KETO MEAL PREP

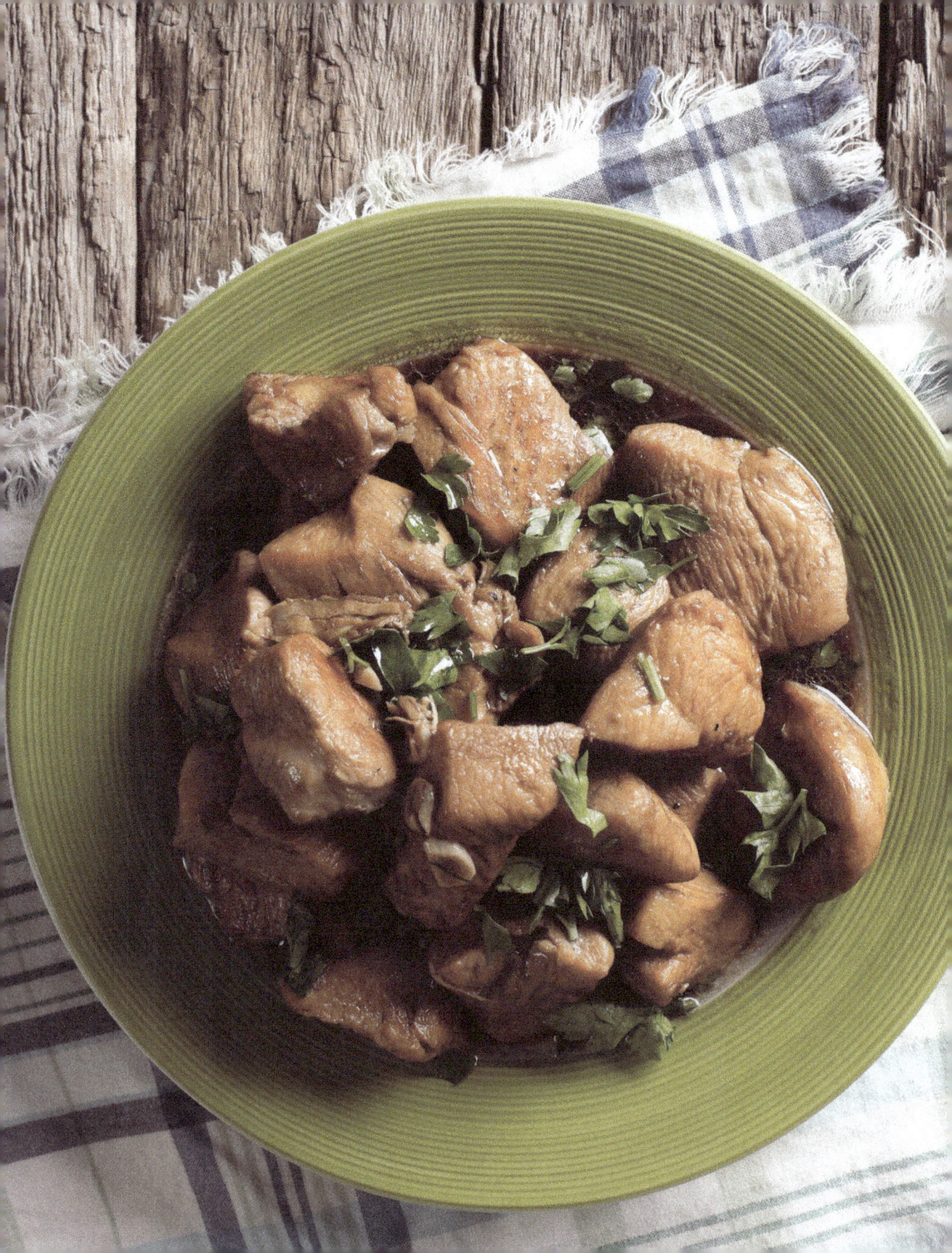

Keto Meal Prep

Essential Ketogenic Diet Meal Prep Guide For Beginners

30 Day Ultra Low Carb Meal Plan to Prep, Grab, and Go

Stephanie Ferrari

Legal Notice

Copyright (c) 2018 Stephanie Ferrari

All rights are reserved. No portion of this book may be reproduced or duplicated using any form whether mechanical, electronic, or otherwise. No portion of this book may be transmitted, stored in a retrieval database, or otherwise made available in any manner whether public or private unless specific permission is granted by the publisher.

This book does not offer advice, but merely provides information. The author offers no advice whether medical, financial, legal, or otherwise, nor does the author encourage any person to pursue any specific course of action discussed in this book. This book is not a substitute for professional advice. The reader accepts complete and sole responsibility for the manner in which this book and its contents are used. The publisher and the author will not be held liable for any damages caused.

Print ISBN/SKU: 9781775274247

E-book ISBN/SKU: 9781775274254

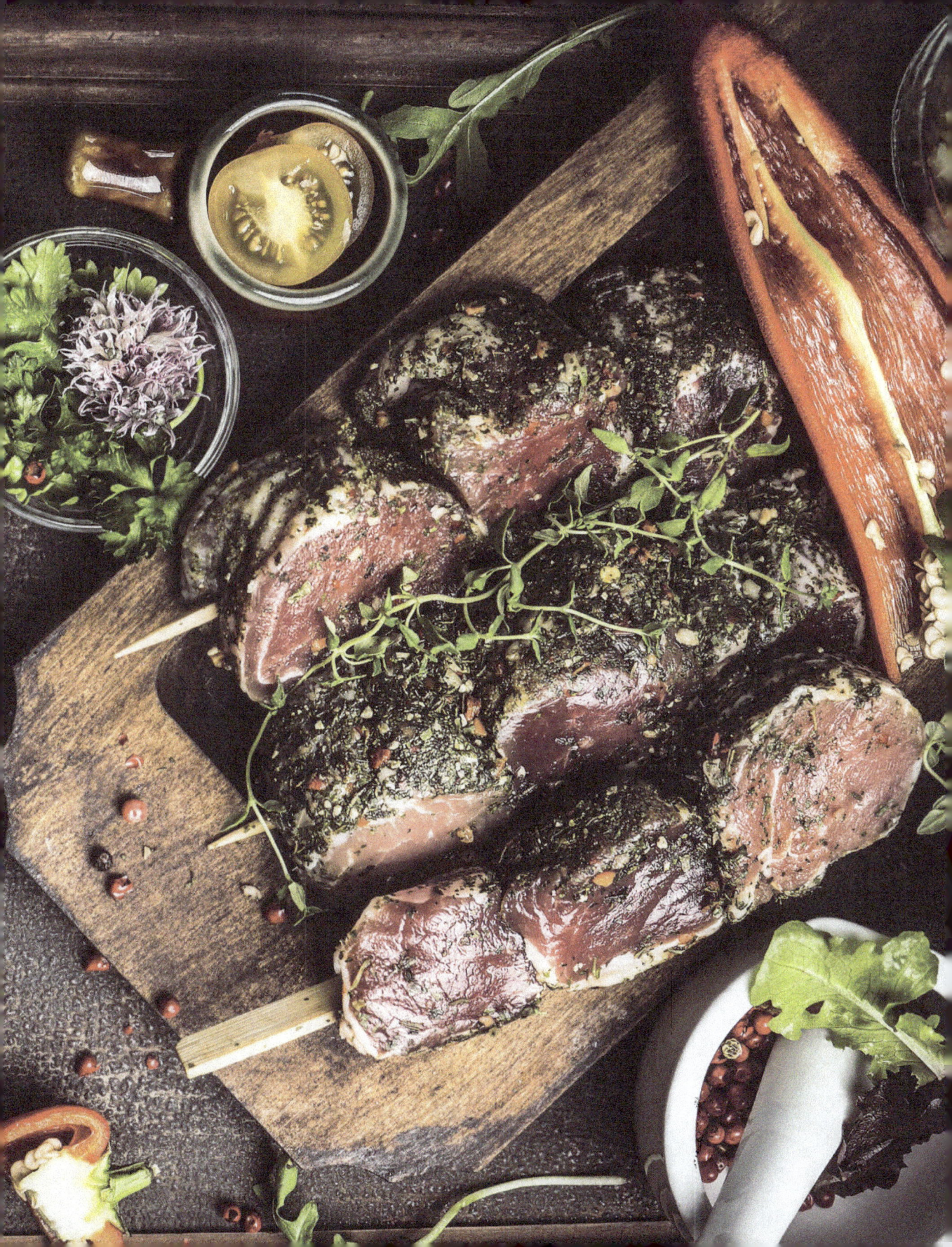

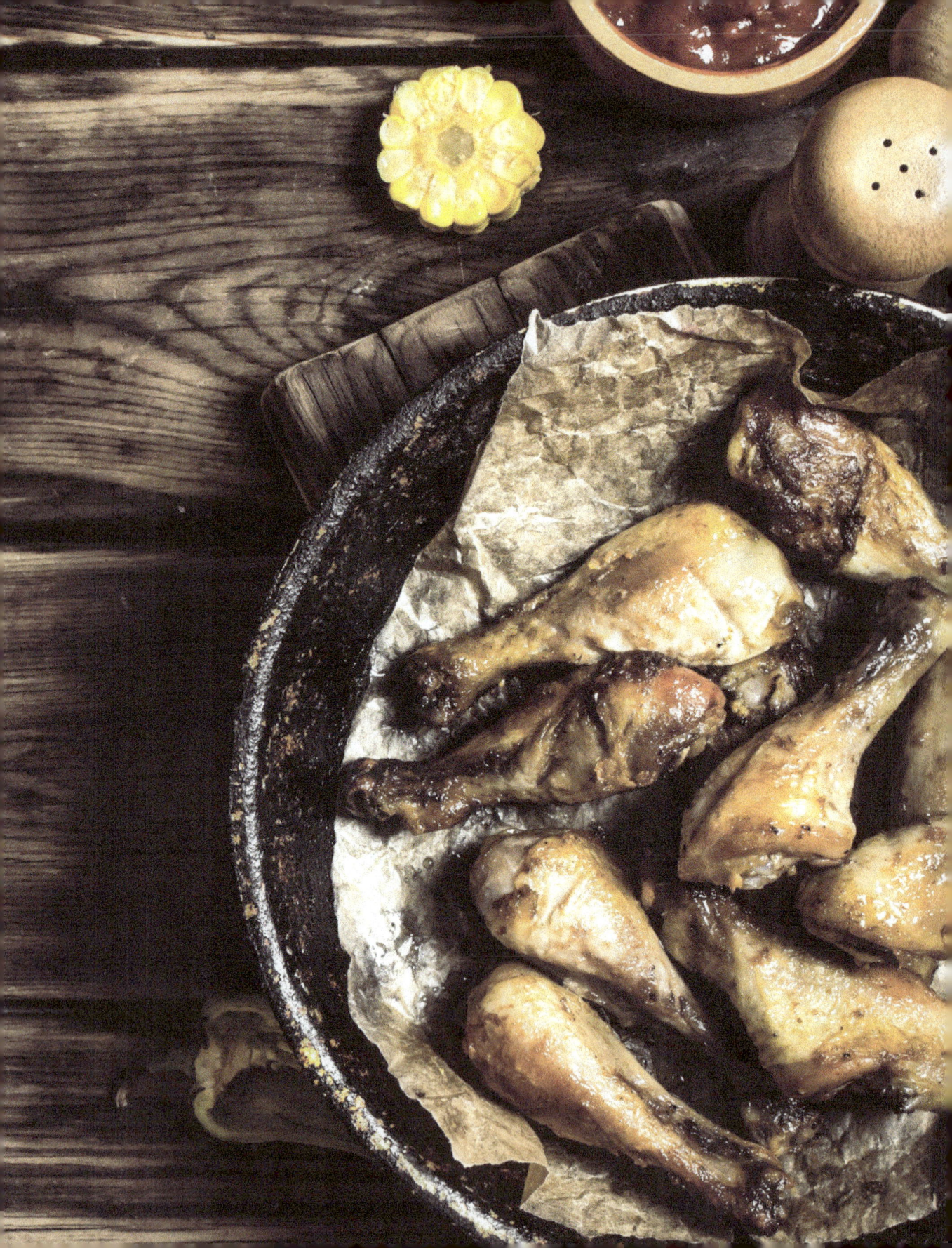

Contents

MY KETO JOURNEY, AS SIMPLE AS PREP, GRAB, AND GO 13

INTRODUCTION 15

CHAPTER 1: KETOGENIC DIET BASICS 17

CHAPTER 2: WHAT TO EAT (AND NOT EAT) 23

CHAPTER 3: EXERCISE AND THE KETOGENIC DIET 29

CHAPTER 4: MEAL PREPPING ON THE KETOGENIC DIET 33

CHAPTER 5: TIPS FOR SUCCESS 37

DAY 1 BREAKFAST: CHORIZO CREPES 44

DAY 1 LUNCH: GRILLED SALMON 45

DAY 1 DINNER: ROASTED CHICKEN 46

DAY 2 BREAKFAST: KETO ALMOND PANCAKES 47

DAY 2 LUNCH: PORK MEDALLIONS 48

DAY 2 DINNER: MEDITERRANEAN-STYLE SALMON 49

DAY 3 BREAKFAST: SAVORY SPINACH CREPES 50

DAY 3 LUNCH: CHEESEBURGER SALAD 51

DAY 3 DINNER: CHICKEN TACO BOWLS 52

DAY 4 BREAKFAST: CINNAMON ROLL PANCAKES 53

DAY 4 LUNCH: PORK "EGG ROLL" BOWLS 54

DAY 4 DINNER: SALMON PATTIES 55

DAY 5 BREAKFAST: BACON MUSHROOM CREPES 56

DAY 5 LUNCH: STUFFED GREEN PEPPERS 58

DAY 5 DINNER: CHICKEN TIKKA MASALA 59

DAY 6 BREAKFAST: RASPBERRY PANCAKES 60

DAY 6 LUNCH: SPINACH AND SALMON SALAD WITH STRAWBERRY VINAIGRETTE 61

DAY 6 DINNER: SLOW COOKER PULLED HAM 62

DAY 7 BREAKFAST: EGG AND SAUSAGE BAKE 63

DAY 7 LUNCH: BEEF WITH ZOODLES 64

DAY 7 DINNER: CASHEW PORK STIR FRY 65

DAY 8 BREAKFAST: RASPBERRY CHEESECAKE SMOOTHIES 66

DAY 8 LUNCH: HAM ROLL-UPS 68

DAY 8 DINNER: CHICKEN BREASTS WITH LEMON DILL BUTTER 69

DAY 9 BREAKFAST: ZUCCHINI AND ONION EGGS 70

DAY 9 LUNCH: BROCCOLI BEEF ALFREDO 71

DAY 9 DINNER: CHICKEN CORDON BLEU CASSEROLE 72

DAY 10 BREAKFAST: BACON CHEDDAR SCRAMBLE 73

DAY 10 LUNCH: HAM AND CHEDDAR CREPES 74

DAY 10 DINNER: GRILLED BURGERS 75

DAY 11 BREAKFAST: TZATZIKI EGGS 76

DAY 11 LUNCH: EGG BITES WITH BACON 77

DAY 11 DINNER: PESTO CHICKEN 78

DAY 12 BREAKFAST: HAM & SWISS FRITTATA 80

DAY 12 LUNCH: WILTED SPINACH SALAD 81

DAY 12 DINNER: PIZZA BURGERS 82

DAY 13 BREAKFAST: BRUNCH MEAT LOAF 83

DAY 13 LUNCH: TUNA SALAD 84

DAY 13 DINNER: TURKEY ZUCCHINI BOATS 85

DAY 14 BREAKFAST: SAUSAGE, EGG & CHEESE SLICES 86

DAY 14 LUNCH: NUTTY SWISS BITES 87

DAY 14 DINNER: AVOCADO EGG SALAD WRAPS 88

DAY 15 BREAKFAST: TURKEY SKILLET 89

DAY 15 LUNCH: CURRY DEVILED EGGS 90

DAY 15 DINNER: HOISIN BURGERS 91

DAY 16 BREAKFAST: SPINACH FRITTATA WITH BACON 92

DAY 16 LUNCH: ASPARAGUS MIMOSA 93

DAY 16 DINNER: COUNTRY-STYLE RIBS 94

DAY 17 BREAKFAST: BACON-WRAPPED SAUSAGE 96
DAY 17 LUNCH: GRILLED CHEESE SANDWICHES 97
DAY 17 DINNER: CREAMY WHITE CHILI 98
DAY 18 BREAKFAST: KETO COCONUT PANCAKES 99
DAY 18 LUNCH: LEMON BUTTER TILAPIA 100
DAY 18 DINNER: PULLED PORK 101
DAY 19 BREAKFAST: KETO VANILLA YOGURT 102
DAY 19 LUNCH: BACON CHEDDAR SANDWICHES 103
DAY 19 DINNER: MEATBALL PARMIGIANA 104
DAY 20 BREAKFAST: PANCAKES WITH PEANUT BUTTER FLUFF 105
DAY 20 LUNCH: TILAPIA CAKES 106
DAY 20 DINNER: SHREDDED PORK TACO SALADS 107
DAY 21 BREAKFAST: CHOCOLATE ALMOND SMOOTHIES 108
DAY 21 LUNCH: HAM AND SWISS PANINI 109
DAY 21 DINNER: MEATBALL STROGANOFF 110
DAY 22 BREAKFAST: BERRIES AND CREAM PANCAKES 111
DAY 22 LUNCH: KALE PESTO TILAPIA 112
DAY 22 DINNER: SMOKY SLOW COOKER CHICKEN 113
DAY 23 BREAKFAST: GREEN SMOOTHIES 114
DAY 23 LUNCH: BUTTERED ZOODLES 116
DAY 23 DINNER: BBQ MEATBALLS 117
DAY 24 BREAKFAST: BACON AND EGG CUPS 118
DAY 24 LUNCH: KETO QUESADILLA 119
DAY 24 DINNER: SMOKY CHICKEN SOUP 120
DAY 25 BREAKFAST: STRAWBERRY CHEESECAKE SMOOTHIES 121
DAY 25 LUNCH: GARLIC SHRIMP ZOODLES ALFREDO 122
DAY 25 DINNER: EGG YOLK FRITTATA 123
DAY 26 BREAKFAST: VEGGIE BACON EGG CUPS 124
DAY 26 LUNCH: AVOCADO SALAD 125

DAY 26 DINNER: BUTTER-ROASTED TURKEY BREASTS 126
DAY 27 BREAKFAST: SMOKED CHICKEN POCKETS 127
DAY 27 LUNCH: ZOODLES WITH THAI PEANUT SAUCE 128
DAY 27 DINNER: TACO BAR 129
DAY 28 BREAKFAST: CHEESY BACON EGG CUPS 130
DAY 28 LUNCH: EGGPLANT TURKEY LASAGNA 132
DAY 28 DINNER: GRILLED COD FILLETS 133
DAY 29 BREAKFAST: COCONUT ALMOND BREAD 134
DAY 29 LUNCH: ZUCCHINI ENCHILADA BAKE 135
DAY 29 DINNER: CUCUMBER SALAD WITH COD AND BASIL 136
DAY 30 BREAKFAST: TOAST WITH ALMOND BUTTER 137
DAY 30 LUNCH: TURKEY PARMESAN 138
DAY 30 DINNER: SLOPPY JOSÉ CASSEROLE 139
REFERENCES AND RESOURCES 140
INDEX 142

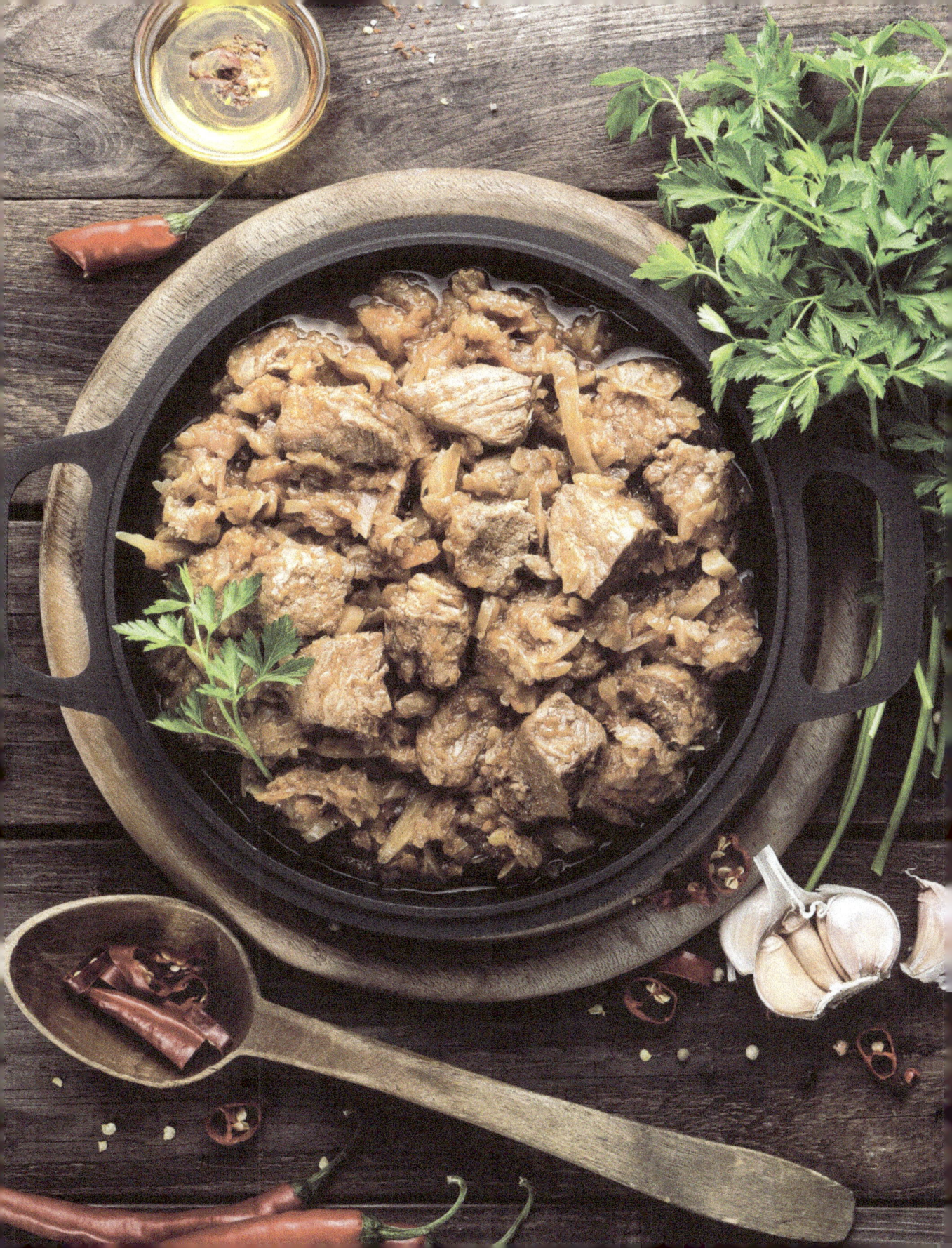

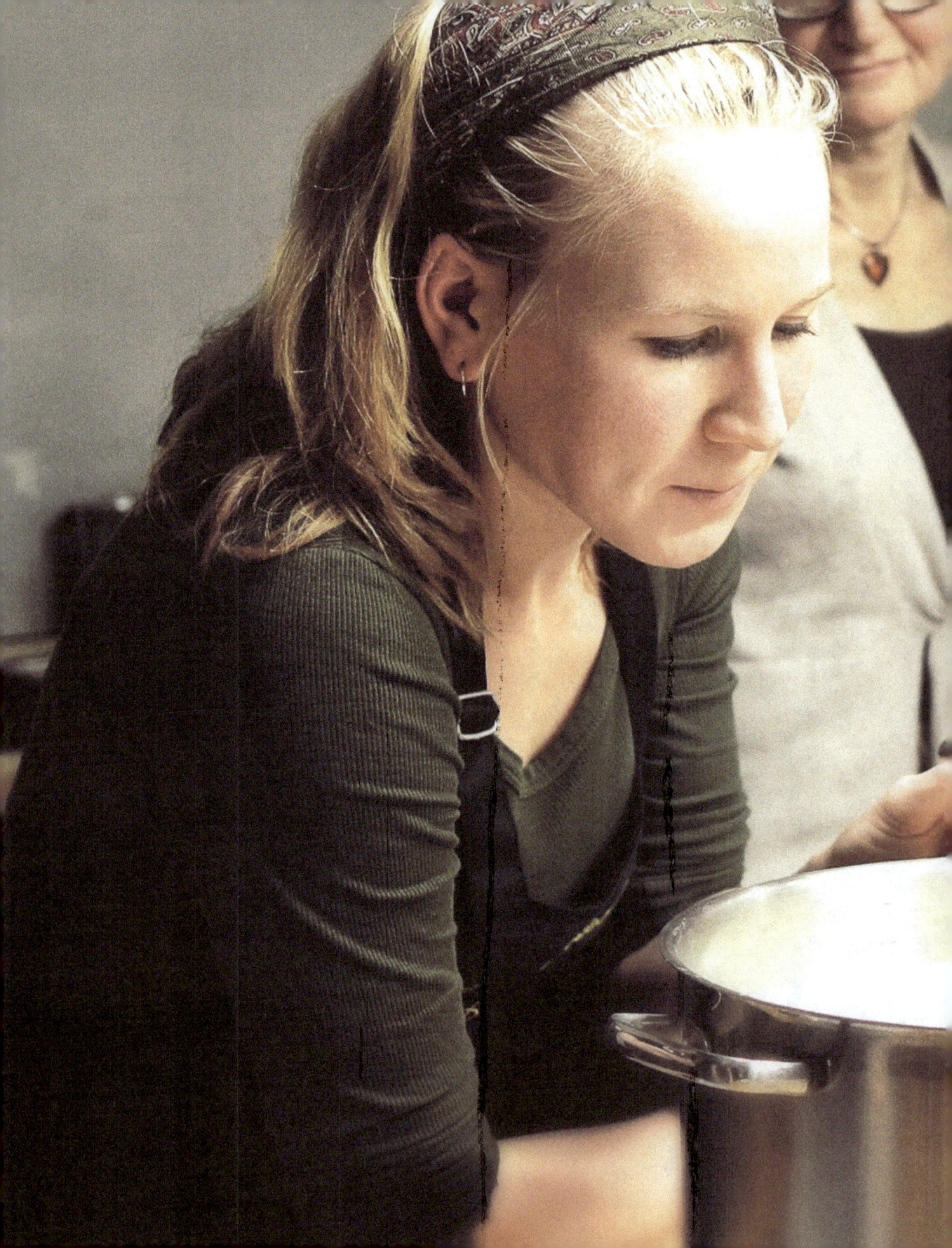

My Keto Journey, as Simple as Prep, Grab, and Go

For years, the majority of my diet consisted of carbs. Pasta, bread, potatoes, pizza... I loved it all. However, I also wanted to lose some weight and improve my health. I frequently struggled with fatigue, brain fog, and just feeling low energy. I knew that my carb-heavy diet was playing a role. I tried some other diets, but when it was when I started getting into the ketogenic diet that my perspective on food completely changed.

Ketosis can seem counterintuitive to the uninitiated. The whole idea that to lose body fat, one has to eat *more* fat may seem implausible at first. But the simple fact is that eating fat isn't the reason why people gain weight. When people eat a lot of carbs, the body turns them into glucose, a useable fuel source. Since I'm not an athlete, most of the glucose I was consuming before I went keto wasn't being used for energy. It was stored as body fat. The fat found in meat, full-fat dairy, oils, and other food doesn't end up stored like that if the body consumes enough. The magic ratio of 60-75% fat and only 5-10% carbs allows the body to enter ketosis, which is when the liver produces ketones during the process of turning fatty acids into a useable fuel source.

Ketones have all kinds of cool health benefits, like clearing up brain fog, protecting the body against disease, and more. To this day, the more I learn about the ketogenic diet, the more convinced I become that this is the way we were meant to eat. Sure, the restrictiveness might make you worry a little if you are just setting out on your keto journey. Some people feel it is hard to give up grains and refined sugars, and I totally get that. But don't worry! It will become clear as you enjoy the recipes in this cookbook that you can still eat a lot of really good food on this diet, which isn't the case for a lot of restrictive eating plans out there.

Since meal-planning is such an important part of any new diet (and the focus of this book), I could see from early on in my keto journey that I would be eating a lot of meals with grass-fed meats, seafood, lots of vegetables, cheese, and other delicious ingredients. By writing lists ahead of time based on the meals I planned on making, getting the right containers, and portioning out food according to the ketogenic guidelines, the diet was not nearly as challenging as I thought it would be. I felt a lot more in control and saw results quicker than I probably would have if I wasn't so organized. I also saved money, which is important for all of us these days.

This book will help you start the ketogenic diet on the right foot. In addition to basic info about what you can and can't eat, you'll learn how exercise fits into the picture and how to prepare for the keto flu, which is common during the first weeks of the new diet. Staying hydrated and eating lots of protein can help make the transition easier. As for long-term success, you should adopt other healthy habits like getting quality sleep and reducing your stress levels. The ketogenic diet isn't merely a "weight-loss diet," it's a diet that can transform every area of your life including your mental health. Meal-planning will make the diet much easier and more effective. Let me be your guide.

With Love,
Stephanie Ferrari

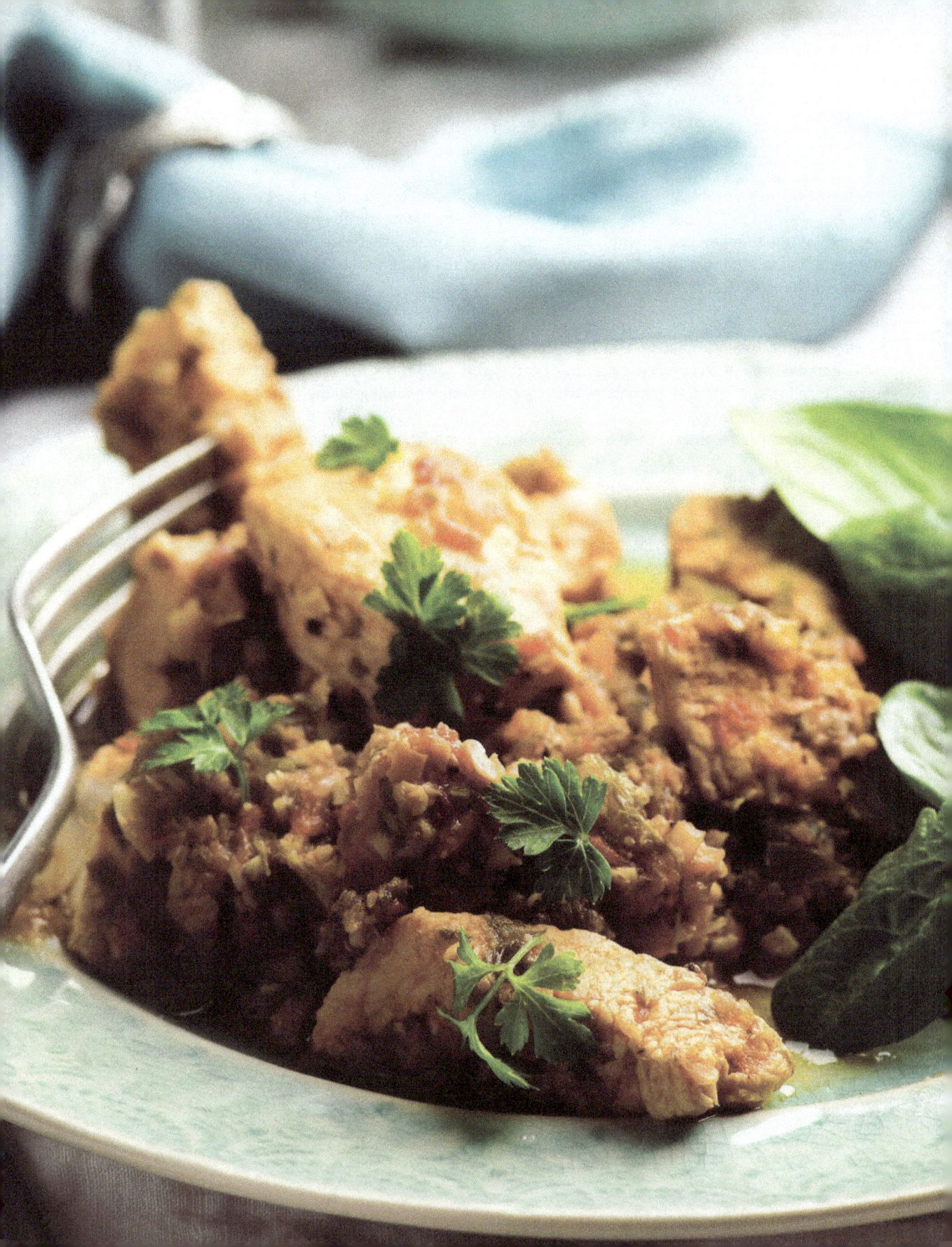

Introduction

Before diving into a new diet, it's always a good idea to learn as much as you can about it. This introduction provides the basics of the ketogenic diet, including its history and the science of ketosis.

You'll learn about the benefits and also the downsides, because no diet is perfect, and it's important to get a comprehensive view of it before making a decision about how best to promote your own health and well-being. You'll also get a thorough rundown of what you're allowed to eat, what is not allowed, and how exercise plays a role in ketosis.

Since this book is primarily about meal prepping on the ketogenic diet, there's also a chapter on why it matters and tips that will make the process easier.

Speaking of tips, how do you succeed on the keto diet in the long-run? You'll learn about getting through the keto flu and ways to stay on track afterwards. With this information, you'll be on a strong footing for success.

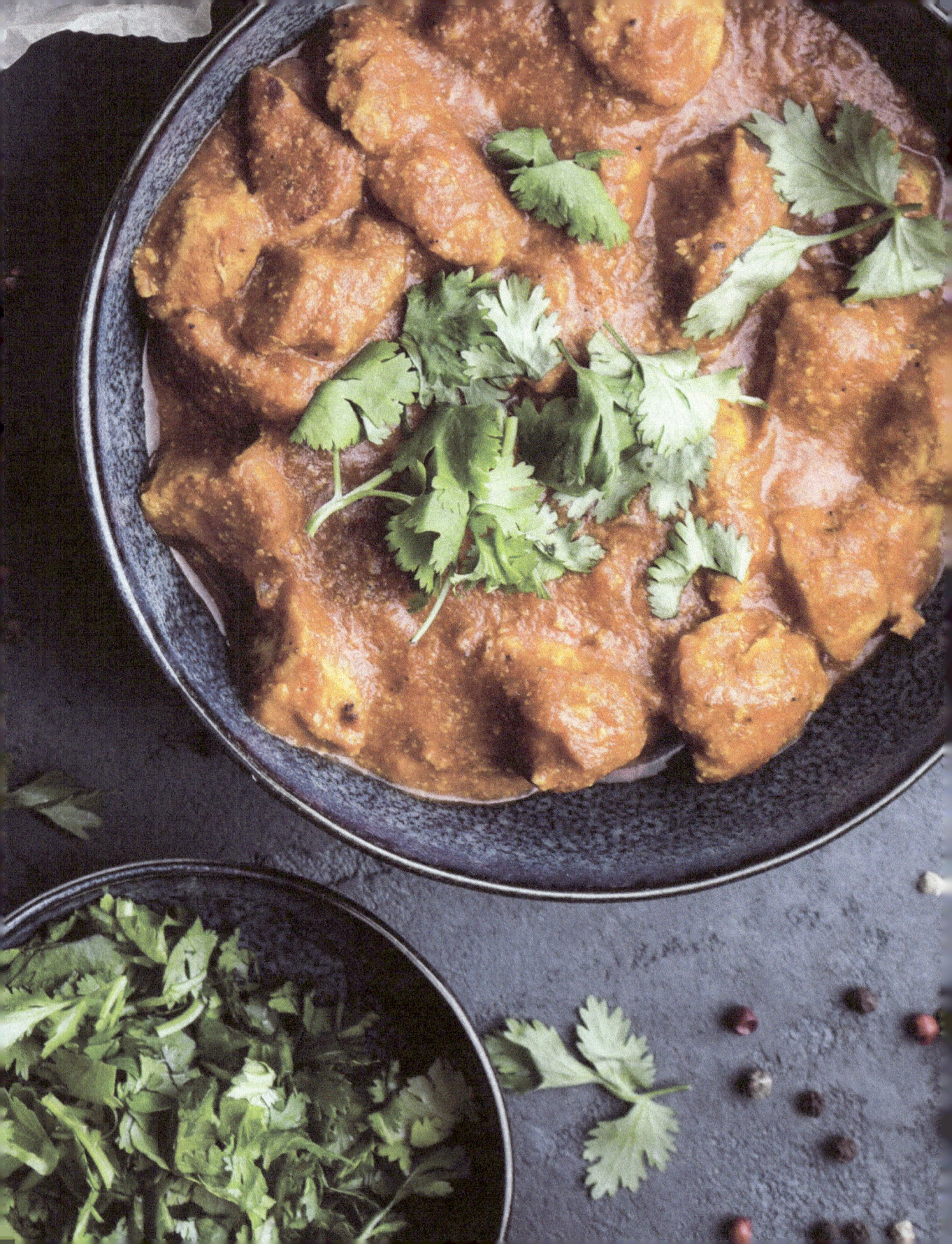

Chapter 1: Ketogenic Diet Basics

The origins of the ketogenic diet can be found in ancient times. Doctors from Greece, Persia, and other countries knew that diet must play a role in treating disease, so they experimented. In 400 B.C.E., Hippocrates is said to have told a patient suffering from seizures to fast. His seizures stopped and Hippocrates began asking all his epileptic patients to intermittently refrain from food. Fasting became the accepted treatment for years.

In 1911, doctors wanted to figure out why exactly fasting worked. They tried asking patients to stop eating meat and eat fewer calories. This also reduced seizures.

In 1921, an endocrinologist studied the role of nutrition again and figured out that a low-carb, high-fat diet had the same effects as fasting. Why? The human liver produces three water soluble compounds (known as ketones) when the person is fasting *or* eating a low-carb, high-fat diet. A high presence of ketones are linked to fewer seizures.

Dr. Russell Wilder from the Mayo Clinic continued researching low-carb, high-fat diets and coined the name "Ketogenic Diet" in 1923. Lots of doctors began prescribing the diet for patients. However, once anti-seizure medications became all the rage, the diet wasn't as popular. In the 1990's, it regained public attention thanks to a Dateline special and made-for-tv movie ("...First Do No Harm") with Meryl Streep.

The low-carb concept was adopted by weight-loss diets like Atkin's as people began reporting other benefits beyond the anticonvulsant effect. This is when the modern low-carb phenomenon really began to catch steam.

Today, the Paleo lifestyle is often linked to the keto diet, though that's mostly just because both diets eliminate grains, processed food, and refined sugar. The keto diet, however, is not based on food availability to paleolithic humans and it emphasizes macronutrients.

How Does The Ketogenic Diet Work?

You know that a ketogenic diet produces ketones, but how? And why does it matter? When you aren't on the keto diet, you probably eat a lot of carbs. Carbs are actually healthy and necessary for life, but we tend to eat way more than we need. The body turns carbs into glucose, which we use for energy. However, if you eat a lot of carbs and don't use all the energy they produce, the excess glucose gets stored as body fat. When you go on the keto diet, you're depriving the body of its usual fuel source. It must switch to fat, which you must eat in abundance. How much fat exactly? Your calories are rationed into fat, protein, and carbs. Every day, the breakdown will be: 60-75% from fat, 15-30% from protein, and 5-10% from carbs.

Remember, fiber carbs don't count toward your carb limit. These are subtracted from your total carb consumption, so you end up with *net* carbs. For most people, they can only eat about 20 net carbs per day on the ketogenic diet. .

To use fat as fuel, the liver has to break it down in a process called "ketosis." During ketosis, the liver also produces ketones, which are used by your mitochondria, muscles, and brain. If your body doesn't need all the ketones it makes, they are eliminated as waste and *not* stored as fat.

How do you know if you're in ketosis or not? At the beginning of your diet, you'll be testing your ketone levels using a urine strip, a breathalyzer, or a blood test. At the start of the keto diet, you lose a lot of ketones through urine because the body hasn't figured out how to use them just yet. We mentioned earlier that there are three types of ketones. Urine strips test for acetoacetate. Breath analyzers measure acetone, which happens to line up pretty accurately with the last type of ketone: beta-hydroxybutyrate. Blood tests test just for BHB.

All three tests will probably measure your ketones in mmol/L or milligrams per decilitre. You are officially in ketosis if you are between 1.5 and 3.0 mmol/L. Anything higher than 3.0 mmol/L doesn't offer additional benefits. Ketones also make the blood more acidic, which can lead to ketoacidosis. For diabetes, ketoacidosis can be fatal, so people with diabetes should stay at or ideally below 1.6 mmol/L.

The ketogenic diet, which was originally developed to prevent seizures, aims to bring the body into ketosis. This is done by eating lots of fat, a moderate amount of protein, and very few carbs.

BENEFITS OF THE KETOGENIC DIET

Why should you consider the keto diet? For many people, the benefits need to be pretty good to justify eliminating grains and paying more for grass-fed meats. Here are the most compelling reasons to make the switch:

Easier weight loss

For years, people believed that fat caused weight gain. However, more research has shown that it's actually sugar and refined carbs that are to blame. When you go on the keto diet, you're cutting out those foods and replacing them with fat. As we mentioned before, any ketones your body doesn't use are excreted and not stored as fat like glucose is.

Weight loss is also easier on the keto diet because overeating isn't as common. High GI carbs get burned up in the body quickly, so you end up feeling hungry shortly after eating. On the keto diet, the carbs you are allowed to eat are all slow-burning. This means your body disperses the energy from them much more evenly, so you stay satisfied for a longer period of time. Vegetables are also full of fiber, which gives you that "full" feeling. If you've been trying to lose weight, going on the keto diet could be the breakthrough you've been looking for.

Boosts your energy

Another benefit of cutting out refined, packaged, and sugary foods is that your energy will improve. High GI foods cause your blood sugar levels to go up and down. When you're eating mostly fat, your body uses the resulting fuel a lot more efficiently, so your energy levels stay even. You won't feel that "carb crash" after a meal or a short time of jittery energy after sugar.

The other reason keto dieters experience more energy is because they're sleeping better. While first in ketosis, you might actually suffer from a little insomnia and interrupted sleep. This is because your body isn't producing as much melatonin and serotonin. However, studies have shown that the ketogenic diet does improve the quality of your sleep long-term. Keto dieters spend more time in REM. If you suffer from insomnia, you can increase your body's melatonin by eating tart cherries, tomatoes, and flaxseeds. Magnesium, calcium, and B6 are also important for sleep.

Sharpens your mind

Carbs have a tendency to produce a "brain fog," which means it's hard to focus for long periods of time. When you cut out most carbs and eat fat, your mental clarity can dramatically improve. Your brain loves ketones, so upping your intake of fat and entering ketosis is going to improve its abilities. This is especially good news for students and others who need to concentrate a lot during the day.

There's also been research that shows that ketones are really helpful for those with neurological diseases like Alzheimer's and Parkinson's. When you have this type of disease, your body can't use glucose efficiently enough. Having ketones in your system takes care of this issue and fills in the gap. Studies have also shown that patients with diabetes experienced improved cognition when in ketosis.

Protects you against disease

The keto diet eliminates a lot of unhealthy food that plays a role in problems like diabetes, heart disease, and more. This is most likely because the diet can help users lose weight and/or maintain a healthy weight, which protects you against a variety of illnesses. Eating nutritionally-dense foods like grass-fed meats and lots of vegetables will also strengthen your immune system, so you aren't as vulnerable to "everyday" illnesses like the flu and common cold.

Speaking of disease, one of the most common problems in today's society is chronic inflammation. This is when your immune system attacks your own cells, leading to joint pain, leaky gut, and more. Studies have shown that inflammation is caused in part by high GI carbs. By eliminating these, your body can finally heal. Foods like dark leafy greens also reduce inflammation while encouraging healing.

> **Benefits of the ketogenic diet include easier weight loss, higher energy levels, improved cognitive function, and protection against disease.**

POTENTIAL PROBLEMS WITH THE KETOGENIC DIET

There are a few key reasons why people hesitate to take on the ketogenic diet. Two of the reasons are relatively subjective and may not be a big enough deal for some people, but the other two are real concerns you should be aware of:

It's too restrictive for the long-term

Because the ketogenic diet cuts out grain, it's considered a restrictive diet. You also can't eat certain vegetables or fruit because of their carb content, *or* packaged foods with refined sugar. That's a lot of food you can't have. While this is a great diet for resetting your health, it can be very challenging for the long-term. Many people don't stay on the diet very long, which can be a problem if they go back to unhealthy eating habits and undo the progress they've made. Other diets that aren't as restrictive may be better for some people.

Getting into ketosis can be a hard transition

Depending on how carb-heavy your diet is, the first few weeks of the keto diet can be very hard. This is due to the "carb flu" or "keto flu," which causes your body to develop flu-like symptoms while it transitions from carbs to fat as fuel. We'll get into more detail about how to manage this, but just know for now that it's a reason some people don't go on the diet. They don't believe there's ever a good time for a 1-2 week period of feeling nauseated, tired, and grumpy.

Micronutrient deficiency is a risk

A big issue that nutritionists have with all restrictive diets is that it eliminates good sources of important nutrients. Whole grains and high GI vegetables provide many of those vitamins and minerals, so if you aren't careful to get those from other foods or take supplements, you can become deficient. The top three gaps: sodium, potassium, and magnesium. You are the highest risk of losing these during the first weeks of the keto diet, since you're losing a lot of water weight. Be sure to stay thoroughly hydrated and eat foods rich in these nutrients the first few weeks of your diet.

It makes you vulnerable to ketoacidosis

It is possible to have too many ketones in your body. Ketones make the blood more acidic, which can lead to ketoacidosis. Symptoms include dehydration, vomiting, extreme thirst, and stomach pains. If untreated, acidic blood damages your kidneys and liver. Diabetics need to be very careful about ketoacidosis because they're especially vulnerable and it can lead to death.

> **When you're in ketosis, you might experience downsides such as micronutrient deficiency and ketoacidosis. The keto diet is also restrictive and can be difficult to transition into.**

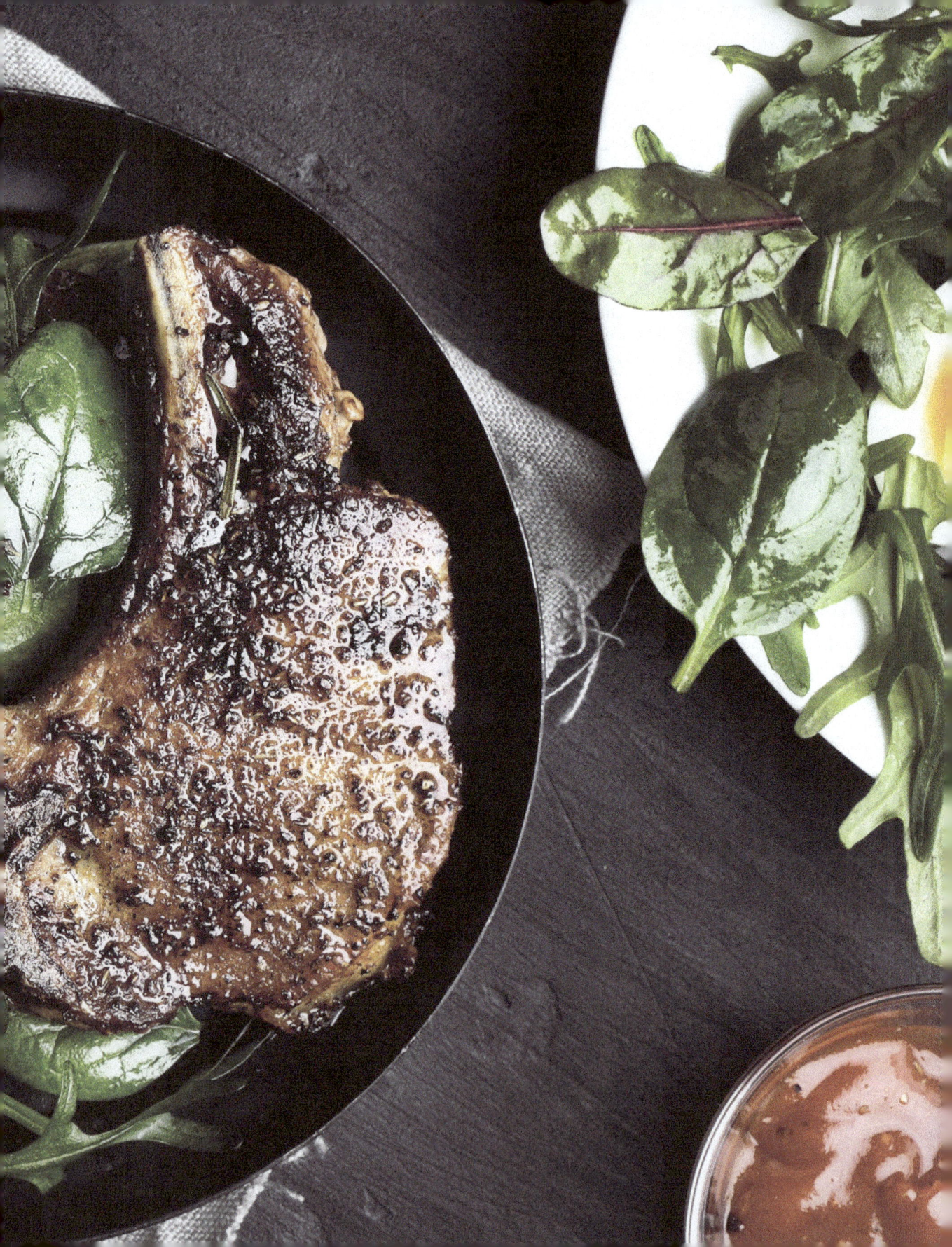

Chapter 2: What To Eat (And Not Eat)

Now that you know what the ketogenic is and how it works, what can you actually eat when you're following the diet? Your two big goals will be getting enough fat and getting enough quality protein. These will come from various oils, nuts, seeds, dairy products, and meat. You also want to eat a lot of vegetables because these are packed with nutrition and fiber, which keeps your digestive system running smoothly. Fruit is not emphasized on the keto diet because most are high on the GI index, but there are some kinds you're allowed to have. This section will also let you know what baking supplies you can use and what beverages you can drink. Lastly, you'll get a list of what you *can't* eat on the ketogenic diet.

FATS

Good sources of fat are the most important part of the ketogenic diet, since they will make up the majority of what you eat. Both monounsaturated and saturated fat are allowed. This list includes the best oils, nuts, seeds, dairy, and fish for fat, but they don't represent all of the nuts/seeds/dairy/fish you can eat. We include separate sections for the rest of those foods.

- Coconut oil
- Coconut cream
- Olive oil
- Avocado oil
- Almond oil
- Grass-fed, full-fat butter
- Duck fat
- Ghee
- Cocoa butter
- Coconut butter
- Unsweetened coconut milk
- Full-fat Greek yogurt
- Avocado
- All-natural unsweetened almond butter
- All-natural unsweetened macadamia nut butter
- Brazil nuts
- Pecans
- Macadamia nuts
- Hemp seeds
- Wild-caught salmon
- Canned (in oil) sardines

PROTEIN

Your body needs quality protein sources for energy as well as cell development and repair. On the keto diet, 15-30% of your calories should come from protein. Here's what you'll be eating:

- Wild-caught seafood
- Shellfish
- Free-range poultry
- Grass-fed beef
- Pasture-raised, organic pork
- Organ meats
- Wild game
- Free-range, organic eggs

VEGETABLES

Pretty much every vegetable is allowed on the ketogenic diet, though you want to choose ones with a low GI index and high nutritional value. Starchy vegetables like potatoes, yams, squash, and more have too many carbs, so they're generally not allowed on the keto diet. You can buy fresh or frozen vegetables; they have the same nutritional value.

- Dark leafy greens
- Cauliflower
- Cucumber
- Celery
- Tomatoes
- Onion
- Bell peppers
- Zucchini
- Broccoli
- Radishes
- Cabbage
- Garlic
- Sea vegetables
- Fermented vegetables

DAIRY

Dairy is a great source of fat and protein on the ketogenic diet. Whatever you get should be full-fat. For the healthiest keto diet, don't overdo it on the cream cheese and cheese, however. Dairy isn't meant to be the main part of your diet. *Note*: No cow's milk allowed on the keto diet, since it's full of sugar.

- Cheddar cheese
- Brie cheese
- Bleu cheese
- Mascarpone cheese
- Mozzarella cheese
- Parmesan cheese
- Swiss cheese
- Ricotta cheese
- Cottage cheese
- Cream cheese
- Greek yogurt
- Heavy whipping cream
- Unsweetened carrageenan-free almond milk
- Unsweetened macadamia nut milk

On the keto diet, you can eat lots of fat; high-quality meat and seafood; low GI vegetables and fruit; full-fat dairy; nuts and seeds; and grain-free, refined sugar-free baking supplies like almond flour and stevia.

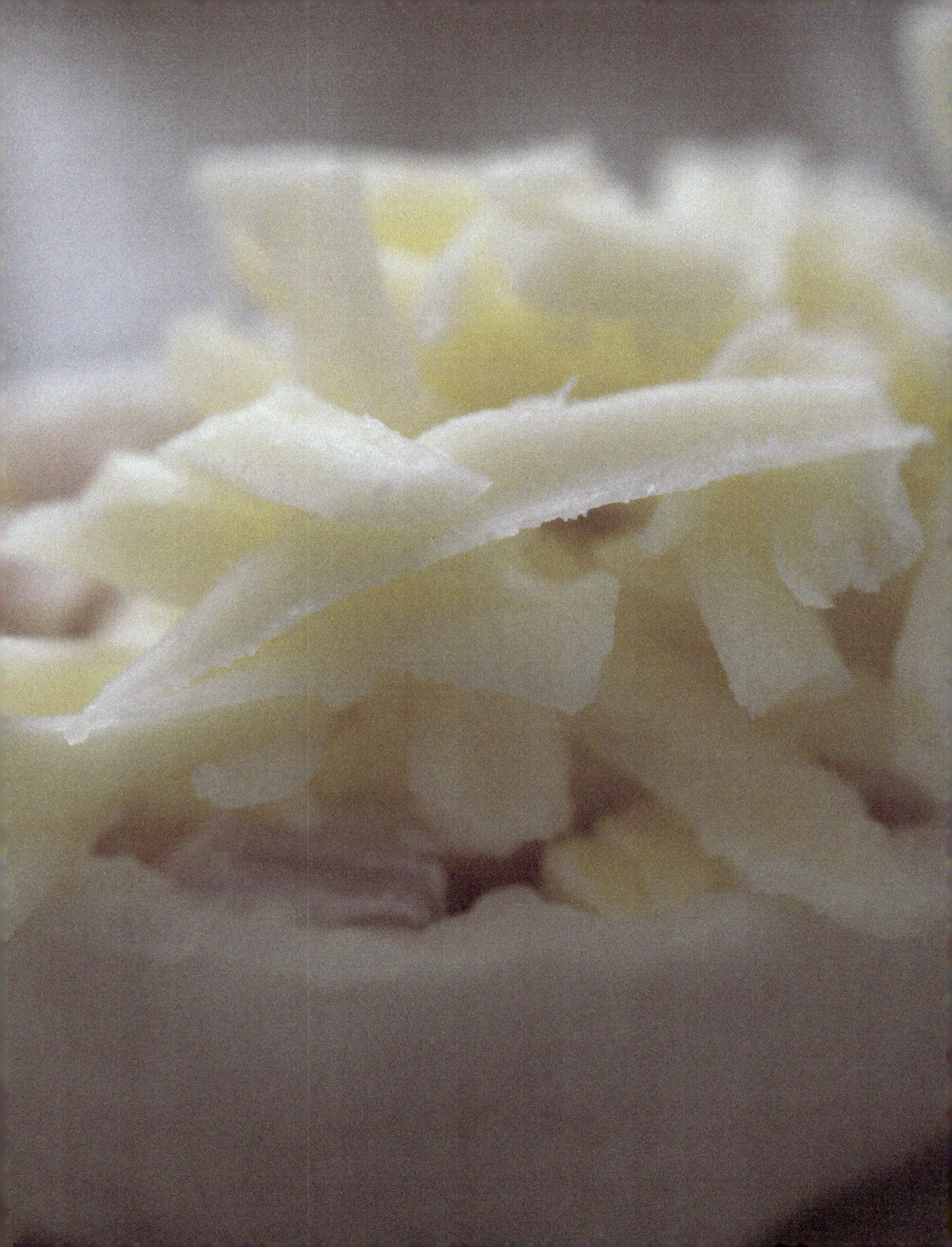

FRUIT

Most fruit contains too many carbs, so you're limited to mostly berries and citrus. Even then, some are higher on the GI scale, so you should eat them rarely. Giving up fruit is often the hardest part for keto dieters.

- Raspberries
- Strawberries
- Blackberries
- Cranberries
- Blueberries (higher on the GI scale)
- Coconut
- Lemons
- Limes
- Peaches (higher on the GI scale)
- Plums
- Oranges (higher on the GI scale)

NUTS/SEEDS

Nuts and seeds are great keto-friendly snacks, but you should avoid eating more than just a handful per day. They have a lot of calories and the carbs can quickly add up. The ones on the "Fat" list that we already named are the best because they have high nutritional value and a low GI. The following are best in moderation:

- Almonds
- Pumpkin seeds
- Sunflower seeds
- Flax seeds
- Chia seeds

BEVERAGES

You can have more than just water on the ketogenic diet, but beverages should contain only natural ingredients and no added sugar. "Diet" sodas, energy drinks, juices, and sweetened teas and coffees are not allowed. Here are your options:

- Water
- Unsweetened herbal tea
- Unsweetened black tea
- Unsweetened coffee
- Sparkling water + seltzers
- Unsweetened coconut water
- Wine (in moderation)

BAKING SUPPLIES

Grain flours are eliminated on the keto diet, but you can use alternative flours and sweeteners. You can also make your own nut and/or seed flours by buying whole nuts and seeds and grinding them into a fine powder. When you're shopping in the baking aisle, here's what you can get:

- Almond flour
- Coconut flour
- Almond meal
- Flax meal
- Psyllium husk
- Baking powder
- Baking soda
- Stevia
- Erythritol
- Stevia/erythritol blends
- Monk fruit
- Natural dark cocoa powder

WHAT YOU CAN'T EAT

The list of what you can't eat on the ketogenic diet is determined by its GI index and fiber content. If a food has a high amount of carbs and not enough fiber to balance it out, it's not allowed. Food might also be eliminated because it's too processed and/or has harmful health effects. Here's what you can't eat on the keto diet:

- All grains
- Beans and legumes
- Starchy vegetables (corn, root vegetables)
- High GI fruit (bananas, apples, mangos, grapes, etc)
- Processed meats
- Low-fat dairy products
- Store-bought condiments
- Most alcohol
- Processed and packaged food
- Sugary treats
- Inflammatory oils
- Natural sweeteners (sugar, maple syrup, corn syrup, agave)
- Artificial sweeteners

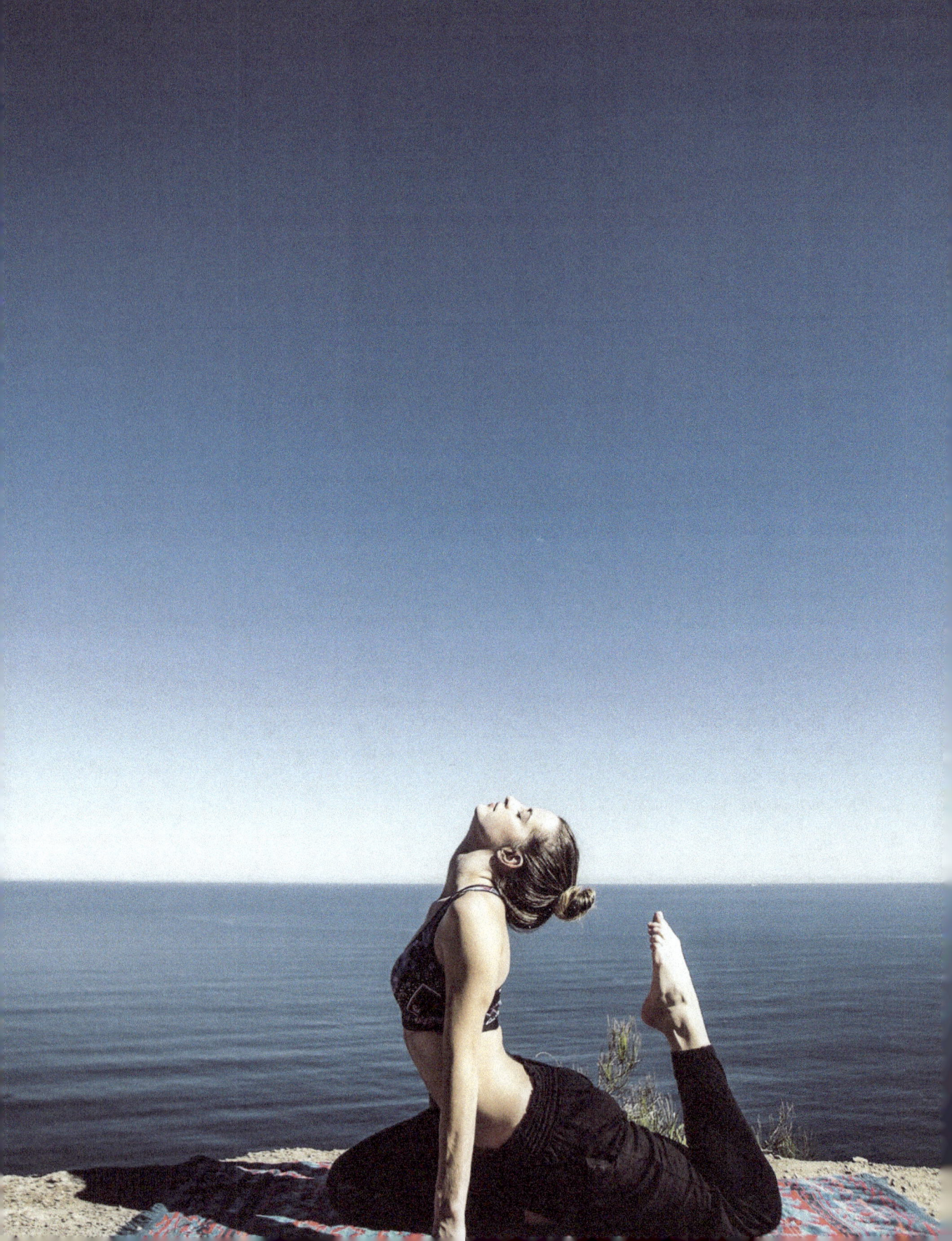

Chapter 3: Exercise And The Ketogenic Diet

How does the keto diet fit into an active lifestyle? Doesn't the body need lots of carbs to fuel intense workouts? Studies have actually shown that the low-carb, high-fat profile of the diet can help endurance athletes so they see better results, more weight loss, and less muscle damage. This chapter digs into why the ketogenic diet is actually one of the best eating plans for active people and how to adjust your activities during the first few weeks of your new diet. Some long-term adjustments are also recommended.

Why Ketosis Benefits Exercise

For years, a high-carb diet was the diet of choice for athletes. This still applies to athletes who engage in high-intensity workouts or anaerobic exercise. Anaerobic exercise includes sports with few breaks (like soccer), sprinting, and heavy weight-lifting. The body prefers carbs. However, for the other types of exercise, the keto diet can be helpful:

Aerobic exercise

Endurance running is a form of aerobic exercise because you don't need quick bursts of speed. A high-fat diet is a good choice and supported by science. A study showed that long-distance runners (going on three-hour runs) who ate a low-carb diet for 20 months burned two to three times more fat than a group who ate the traditional high-carb diet.

Stability exercise

Balance and core strength are essential. People do stability exercises (like exercise balls) when they want to strengthen specific muscle groups and keep their body aligned. The keto diet provides enough energy for low-intensity stability workouts.

Flexibility exercises

These activities are about strengthening your muscles and joints. Yoga is the best example of this type of workout. Because it's low-intensity, your body uses fat for fuel. The keto diet can also help if you experience joint inflammation.

> **Certain forms of exercise are better on the ketogenic diet than others. Endurance training (long-distance running, cycling) and core/flexibility workouts (yoga, pilates, exercise balls) can use fat instead of carbs for fuel, so the keto diet is a good fit.**

THE TRANSITION

Studies show it takes about five weeks for an active person to get back to their normal performance after going on the keto diet. You should take it easy for a while and not push yourself too hard. Engage in more aerobic, stability, and flexibility exercises. Some resistance training is also okay. Expect to feel more fatigued and weaker during these first workouts. If you feel tempted to stop exercising all together, resist. Mild exercise actually helps the ketosis process kick in. Because your body is losing a lot more water and electrolytes than usual, be sure to stay hydrated and get electrolytes from foods like coconut water, fresh citrus juice, and sea salt.

ADJUSTING YOUR KETO DIET FOR AN ACTIVE LIFESTYLE

If you're very active, you will probably have to adjust the keto diet to make the most of its benefits. Tweaking the diet to fit isn't cheating; it prevents injury and ensures that you're getting the fuel you need. The specific changes depend on your exercise goals.

GOAL: GAIN MUSCLE	GOAL: LOSE WEIGHT	GOAL: IMPROVE ENDURANCE
Eat an extra 250-500 calories (mostly fat) per day	Cut down on fat so you reduce calories by 250-500 calories a day	Eat less than 35 grams of carb per day
Eat 1 gram of protein per pound of your bodyweight	Keep eating 1 gram of protein per pound of your bodyweight	If your performance drops, add more carbs *or* add MCT oil to your diet before workouts

Cardio Workouts On The Keto Diet

You know that higher-intensity training isn't a natural fit for the keto diet, but if you want to do that kind of workout, it is possible. You just have to add some extra carbs to your diet and eat them *before* a workout. Around 30 minutes before, eat 15-30 grams of a fast-burning carb like a banana or other fruit. This will give you the burst of energy you need. After the workout, eat another 15-30 grams so your muscles can recover.

The keto diet can be tweaked to provide the best macros for exercise goals like muscle gain, weight loss, and so on.

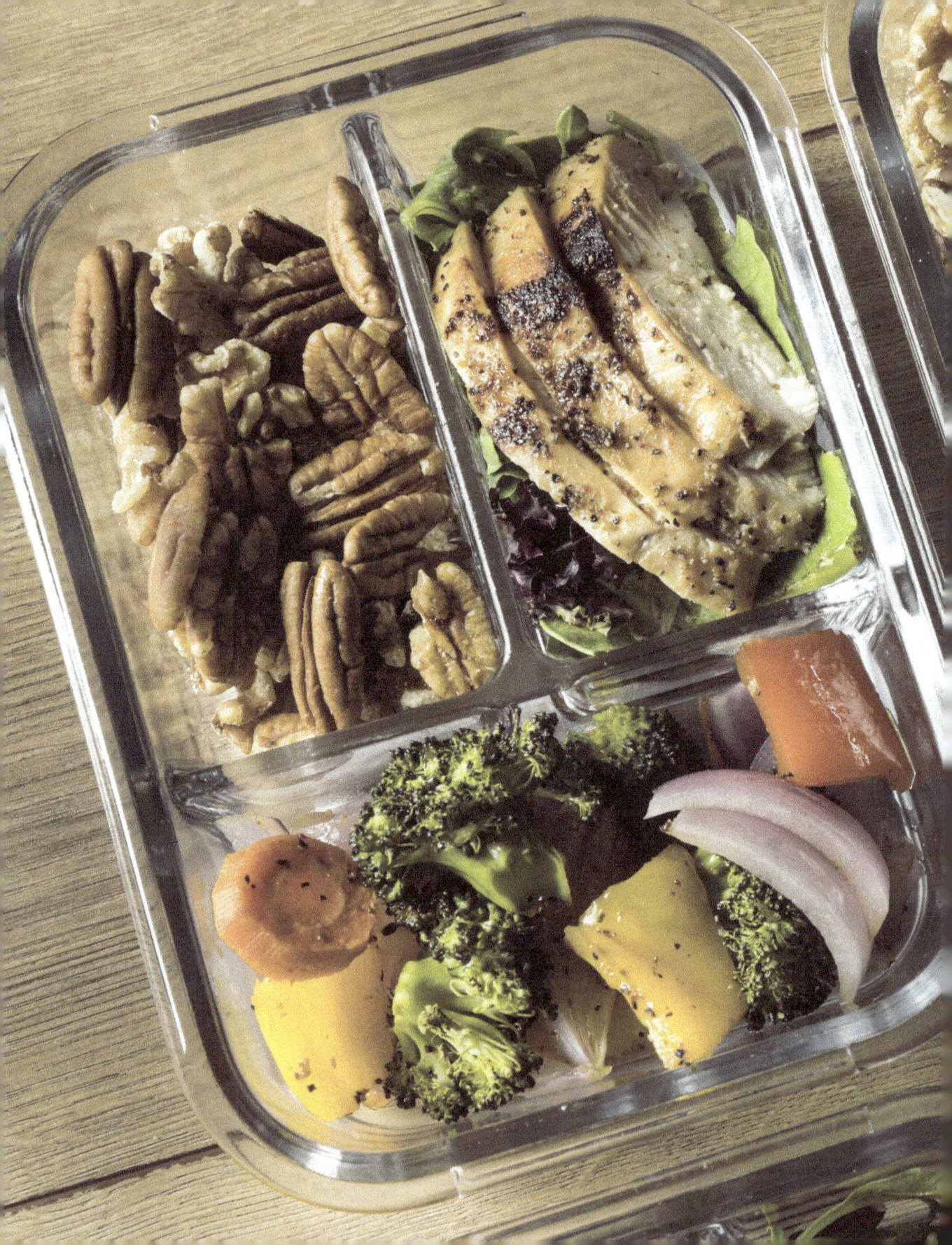

Chapter 4: Meal Prepping On The Ketogenic Diet

Most of us can't spend hours in the kitchen cooking. We need recipes that are fast, easy, and nutritious. The secret to keto-friendly cooking that doesn't burn up time and energy is to meal plan.

This chapter explains the basic why's and how's of meal-planning on the ketogenic diet. Using what you learn in this chapter will give you a powerful "action-plan" for implementing the ketogenic diet in your own life so you can easily enjoy its many benefits. Lots of people think "going keto" is hard. The truth is it can be as easy as *prep, grab, and go*.

BENEFITS

Why is meal-planning so important? There are four main reasons:

Going grocery shopping is easier

You probably write a list before you go shopping, but if you haven't planned out what meals you're going to eat that week, that list might not be enough. How many times have you decided on a dinner and then realized you don't have all the ingredients?

When you plan ahead, you can write down all the ingredients you'll need and then hit up the store. The trip will be quicker, too, then if you were standing in an aisle trying to think of what meals you're going to make.

You can create more interesting meals

With lots of food eliminated on the ketogenic diet, it's easy to fall into a routine where you make boring meals. If you plan, however, you can experiment with different spices, herbs, vegetables, and so on to create more unique meals.

A big part of meal-planning is researching recipes online and in cookbooks (like this one!), which expands your cooking range and bevvy of meal staples. Keeping things interesting on the keto diet is very important if you hope to stay faithful to it in the long-run.

You save money

Grass-fed meats and organic produce aren't cheap. When you meal plan, you can cut down on unnecessary expenses by organizing what you buy, where you buy, and when you buy it. Be on the lookout for sales, frequent grocery stores with good deals, and plan lots of meals with vegetable proteins or meals with smaller amounts of meat.

The keto diet doesn't have to be a lifestyle just for people who make a certain income. Meal-planning can help save you money.

It's easier to get the nutrition and percentages you need

The keto diet is all about percentages of fat, protein, and carbs. You also need to be aware of your nutrition intake because the keto diet cuts out a lot of nutrient-rich foods like grains and beans.

Planning your meals allows you to be more in control about where your calories are going. A big part of meal-planning is working ahead, as well, so you can make meals a few days in advance and know that they each contain the fat and protein you need to stay in ketosis.

You don't have to worry about tracking carbs and fat every single meal time because you already did that work in advance.

> **Benefits of meal-planning include saving money, easier shopping trips, and both interesting and healthy meals.**

TIPS FOR MEAL-PREPPING

What are some specific meal-prepping methods that make the ketogenic diet easier?

Use the right equipment

Don't underestimate the practicality and beauty of a good appliance. Slow cookers let you cook large meals with very little hands-on work, while blenders are great for sauces, smoothies, and more.

You also want really good containers that are easy to wash and durable. If you really want to embrace meal-prep, consider getting a multi-cooker or Instant Pot. You'll get a pressure cooker, rice cooker, slow cookers, and more in just one device.

Always make enough for leftovers

No matter what diet you're on, it's always a good idea to make big batches of every meal. You save time and energy, which is super important on the keto diet since you'll be doing most if not all of your cooking at home.

Take any opportunity you can to work less. The leftovers of these big batches can be eaten as lunches and dinners, or as parts of new meals. If you make more than you can eat in the next few days, freeze it. You can find lots of keto meals designed to be "batched" and freezer-friendly.

Work ahead on recipes that take more work

Lots of people take one day a week to do a lot of meal-prepping. Sunday is a common day, because it's before the chaos of the work week and it gives you Saturday to relax and have fun. On this prep day, take a look at the meals you've planned and work on the ones that take the most time and energy. Meals that can sit in the fridge (think chilies and stews) are good candidates, whereas meals with fresh vegetables will most likely need to be prepped the day of.

Portion ahead of time

If you do nothing else on prep day, you should portion your meals (and snacks, ideally). This might just mean separating out raw chicken breasts into their own freezer bags with some herbs, but anything that saves time is a good idea.

This is also the time when you want to be aware of macronutrients. Every keto meal should consist of mostly fat with a good protein source and as few carbs as possible.

Portion your meals using your percentages, so that's one less thing you have to do when it's time to finish making the recipe.

> **When it comes to meal-planning on the keto diet, actions like using the right containers, making big batches, and portioning in advance can make the diet a lot easier.**

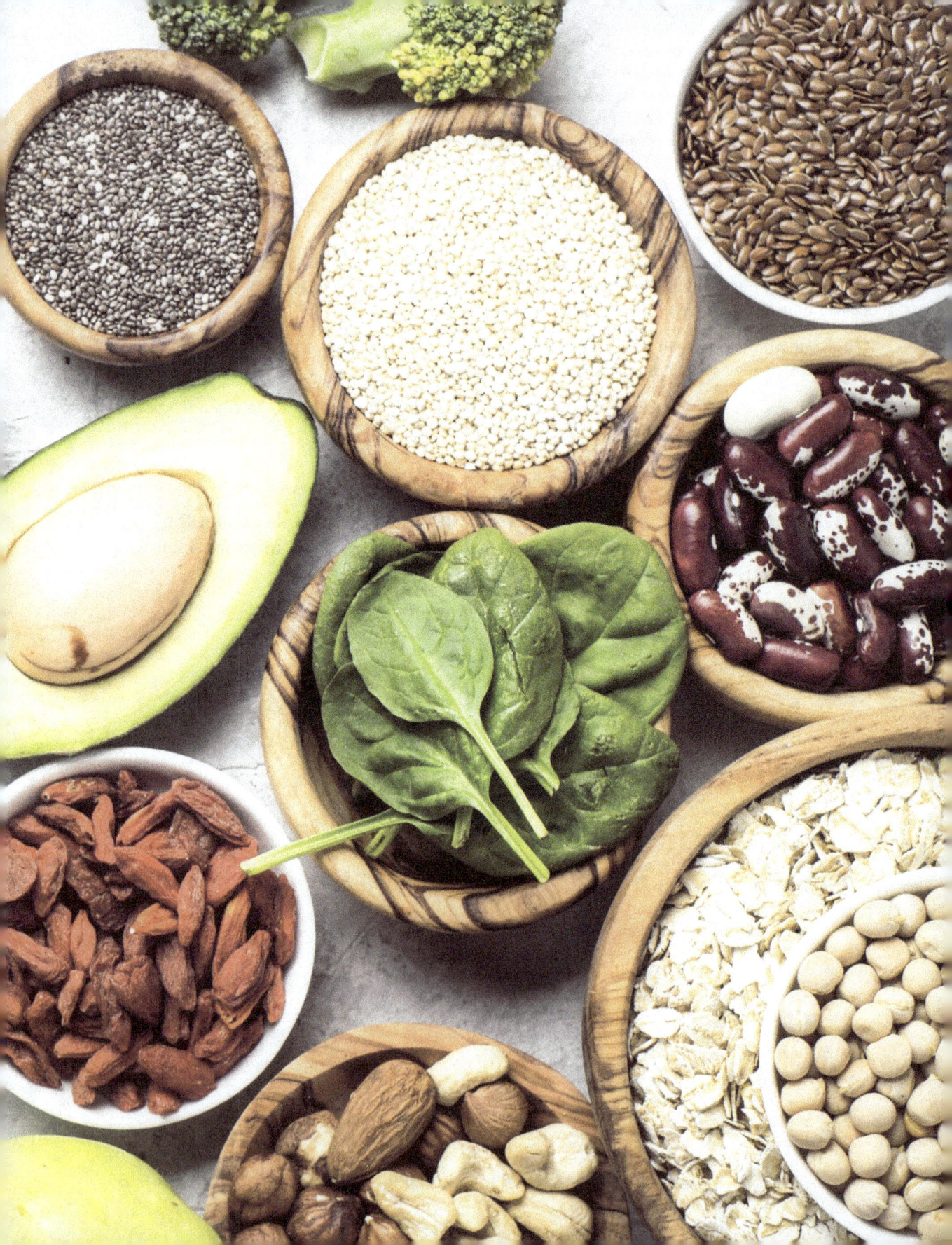

Chapter 5: Tips For Success

How do you stick to the ketogenic diet and enjoy the benefits? This chapter covers how to begin the diet and maintain it for the long haul.

A change in diet can be transformative, so you want to start on the right foot and follow the tips that will make overcoming challenges easier.

What To Do First

You know the basics of the ketogenic diet and how exercise will fit into your new diet. What should you do first? Step 1 is to do an overhaul of your kitchen and stock up on the keto essentials. These are what you always need on hand regardless of your meal plan for that week. Here's a sample list:

- Ground grass-fed beef
- Frozen fish fillets
- Canned tuna
- Bone broth
- Organic chicken (your favorite cut)
- Coconut oil
- Full-fat coconut milk
- Grass-fed butter
- A hard full-fat cheese
- Unsweetened nut milk
- Frozen berries
- Avocados
- Dark leafy greens
- Cucumbers
- Garlic
- Onions
- Tomatoes
- Unsweetened nut butter
- Whole pecans
- Almond flour
- Dry herbs + spices
- Baking powder
- Natural sweetener of some kind
- Dark baking chocolate

Once you have your pantry stocked and all the non-keto foods removed, step 2 is to figure out what your macros are going to be. There are lots of keto calculators online that use information like your weight, health goals, and activity level to give you the specific number of grams of protein, fat, and carbs you'll be eating. Now is also the time to get a ketone reader of some kind so you can track your ketosis progress.

Step 3 is to begin planning out your meals for the first few weeks of your new diet. Look in this cookbook and other resources like recipe blogs to figure out what you want to eat.

Choose meals that are simple, easy to cook in large batches, and meet your nutritional goals. It's a good idea to plan ahead at least three weeks of your main meals, because once you start on the keto diet, you might experience what's known as the keto flu.

To start the keto diet on the right foot, turn your kitchen into a keto-friendly space, determine what your macros will be, and meal-plan for the first few weeks.

What Is The Keto Flu?

When you make a quick shift into the keto diet and cut out a lot of carbs at once, you most likely will experience flu-like symptoms such as headaches, sluggishness, constipation, and so on. Why? The body is making significant changes to use fat instead of carbs for fuel. It's working a lot harder than usual, losing more water, and not getting as much fiber. For most people, the keto flu lasts a week or so, but in the worst cases, it can go on for a month. The severity of symptoms also varies person by person. If you eat lots of refined sugar and carbs, your withdrawal will be worse. What can you do to make the transition easier?

Stay hydrated

When your body moves into ketosis, you lose a lot of water weight. You need to replace that or you'll get dehydrated. Drink more than you would normally. When you get sick of water, sip on keto-friendly beverages like unsweetened coconut water. Bone broth is also a good drink during this time since it's full of nutrition.

Add MCT oil

One way to reduce your symptoms is to speed up the ketosis process. You can do that with MCT oil, or medium-chain triglycerides. These are found in coconut oil, so mix a teaspoon or two into a glass of water every morning. This should help jumpstart the ketosis process.

Eat protein aplenty

When you're starting on the keto diet, don't worry too much about your protein macros. It's better to eat more than you will once you're in ketosis because it keeps you full and energized.

Most people will experience the keto flu during the first week or so of the ketogenic diet. To fight symptoms like headaches and fatigue, be sure to stay hydrated, eat lots of protein, exercise, and consume some MCT oil. If your symptoms are really bad, add some healthy carbs back into your diet until you've transitioned.

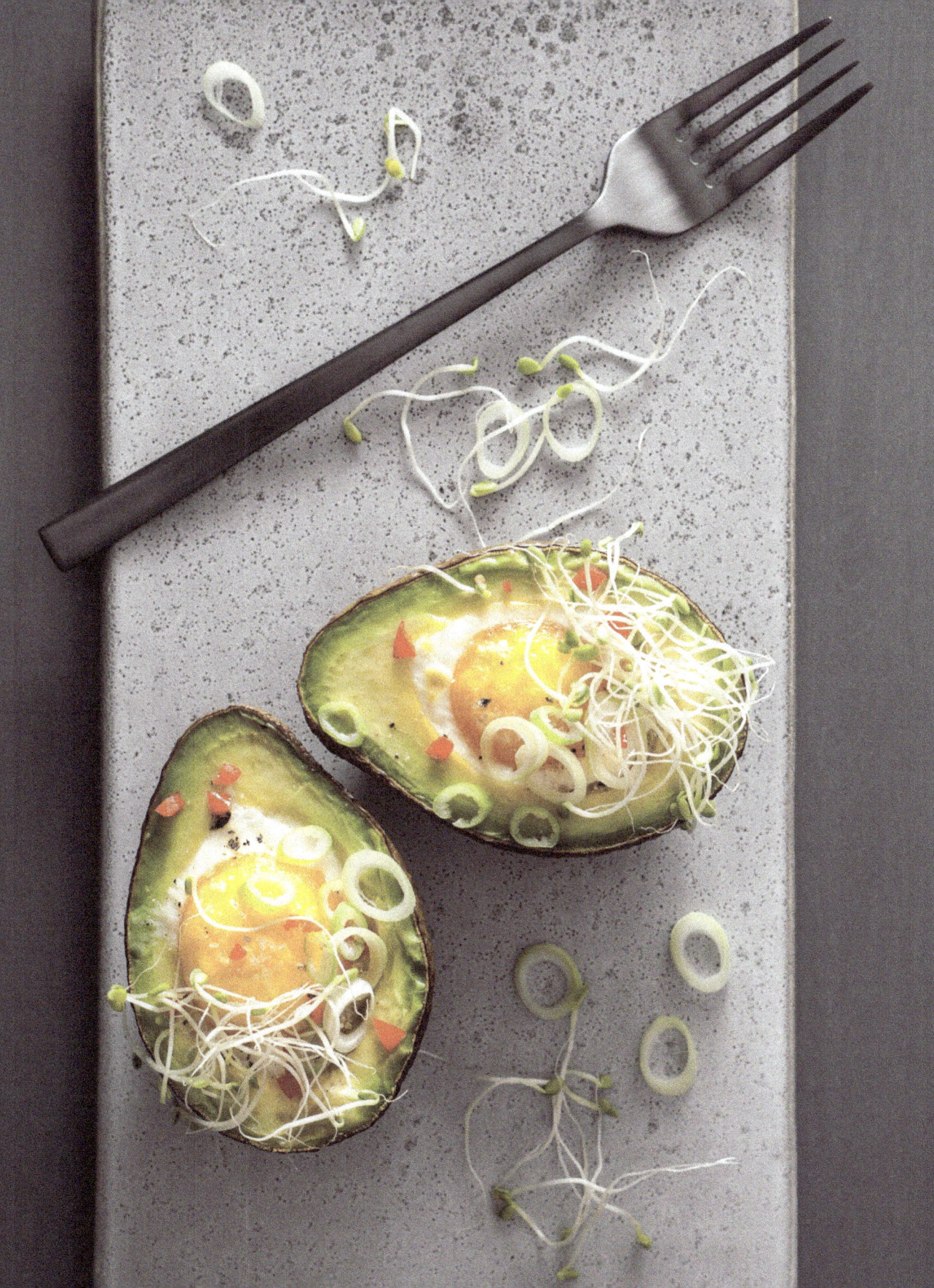

Do some easy exercises

Exercise speeds up ketosis, especially workouts that rely on fat and not carbs for energy. Do some light cardio and yoga. This will get you into ketosis faster and end your keto-flu symptoms.

Eat some healthy slow-burning carbs

If your keto-flu symptoms are worse than you expected, you can slow down your transition. Eat some slow-burning carbs like sweet potatoes, grapes, or nectarines. These are on the high end of the GI index, but still healthy. It will take you a bit longer to get into ketosis, but you'll feel a lot better.

TIPS FOR LONG-TERM SUCCESS

Once you're past the keto flu and in ketosis, there are some other tips that can keep you on track. The keto diet isn't the hardest diet you can go on, but it does have its challenges. Here are ways to ensure you stay healthy and enjoy the most benefits:

Remember electrolytes

On the keto diet, you are more likely to lose electrolytes because the body doesn't hold on to water as much. While this reduces bloating, the lost electrolytes can cause other problems. What are electrolytes exactly? They are minerals that keep your body functioning properly. There are four you should be sure to get through your meals or supplements if necessary.

Sodium - Helps muscle and nerve function/Get through high-quality salt

Calcium - Necessary for blood clotting and strong bones/Get through full-fat dairy and dark leafy greens

Magnesium - Helps strengthen immune system and nerve function/Get through nuts and dark leafy greens

Potassium - Helps fluid balance and blood pressure/Get through avocados, nuts, and dark leafy greens

Maintain a food journal

To keep track of your macros, you'll need to keep a food journal. There are lots of app options like MyFitnessPal that divide up what you ate per day into macros, subtract calories you lost during exercise, and subtract fiber from total carbs.

Educate yourself on impact and low-impact carbs

Even though you're severely restricting your carbs on the ketogenic diet, carbs are not evil. Your body needs them to survive. Know the difference between impact carbs, which affect your blood sugar, and low-impact carbs, which don't. "Impact" is basically another word for carbs with a high GI index. These are the ones you want to avoid. Low-impact carbs are the ones that digest slowly, like dark leafy greens, and provide energy over a longer period of time. These are the ones you *want* to eat.

> **How do you succeed on the ketogenic diet for the long-term? Be sure to keep an eye on your electrolytes, keep a food journal, know the difference between "good" carbs and "bad" carbs, sleep well, and keep your stress levels low.**

Get good sleep

If you're on the ketogenic diet and not getting quality sleep, you won't see a big difference in your health. Good sleep is essential to your overall health, so it needs to be a priority. Aim for an interrupted 8 hours per night in total darkness, so your body can produce the melatonin it needs to stay rested. Before bed, try to begin the winding-down process about an hour before light's out. You can find lots of tips on "sleep hygiene" online if you struggle with insomnia or restlessness.

Reduce your stress

Stress is poison to the body. It can even cut years off your life. This tip doesn't just apply to the ketogenic diet, it's one that everyone should remember. If your life revolves around a stressful job, it's time to make a change. Reconsider your priorities. Do you work to live or live to work? Why? Do you believe more money will make you happy? How much time do you spend doing what you really love? How much time do you spend with your family and friends? Even if you do nothing else, reducing your stress can have a dramatic impact on your health.

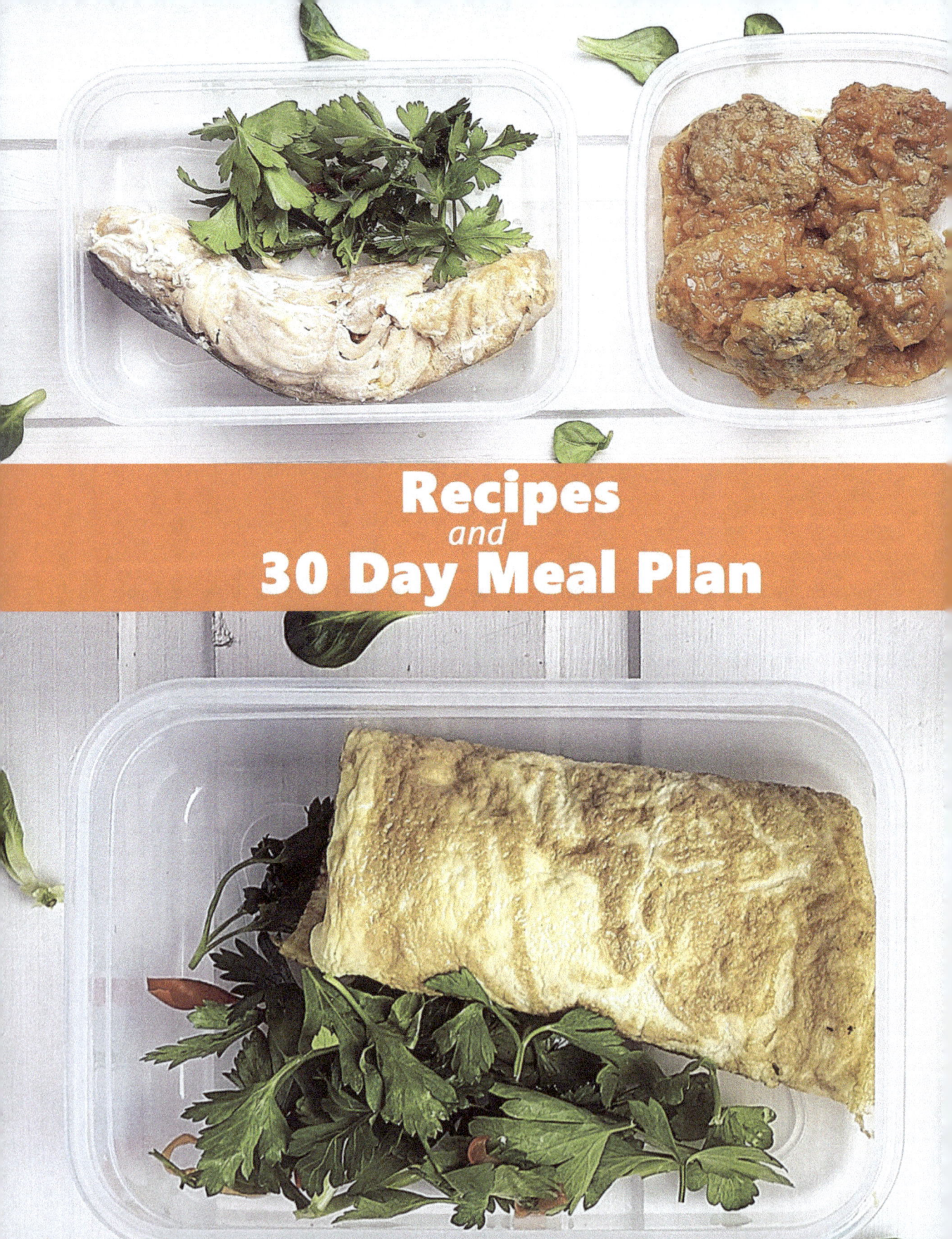

Recipes
and
30 Day Meal Plan

Make your keto journey
as simple as
Prep, Grab, and Go!

Day 1 Breakfast: Chorizo Crepes

Serves: 4 (plus 2 leftover portions) / Preparation time: 10 minutes / Cooking time: 20 minutes

For a spicier garnish, use cayenne pepper instead of the chili powder in the guacamole for these crepes.

12 eggs (lightly beaten)

1/2 cup heavy cream

Salt and freshly ground black pepper, to taste

2 tablespoons butter (plus more as needed)

1 chorizo sausage (about 4 ounces)

1 garlic clove (minced)

1 avocado (halved, pitted)

1 tablespoon chopped fresh cilantro

1 lime (zested, juiced)

Chili powder, to taste

1/2 cup (2 ounces) shredded cojack cheese

1/4 cup sour cream

- In a large bowl, whisk eggs and cream and season to taste with salt and pepper. Melt about 1 teaspoon butter in a medium nonstick skillet over medium heat and fry egg mixture into 12 crepes. Set finished crepes aside and keep warm.

- Remove casing from chorizo if necessary and discard. Crumble sausage into skillet with garlic and cook through over medium heat, stirring frequently. Drain sausage as necessary and set aside.

- For the guacamole, mash avocado flesh and mix with cilantro, lime juice and lime zest. Season guacamole to taste with salt, pepper and chili powder and set aside.

- To assemble, spread chorizo mixture on 4 of the crepes, sprinkle with shredded cheese and roll up to cover filling. Top crepes with guacamole and sour cream and serve immediately. Set remaining 8 crepes aside until cool, cover and refrigerate for later use. Enjoy!

PER SERVING: Calories: 399; Fat: 34g; Protein: 18g; Carbs: 6g; Fiber: 3g Net Carbs: 3g; Fat 77% / Protein 22% / Carbs 1%

Day 1 Lunch: Grilled Salmon

Serves: 2 (plus 3 leftover portions) / Preparation time: 10 minutes / Cooking time: 8 minutes

For a complete meal, brush fresh asparagus spears with olive oil, season to taste with salt and pepper and roast on the grill alongside the salmon until tender, 2 to 3 minutes.

8 skin-on salmon fillets (about 8 ounces each)   1/2 teaspoon salt, plus more to taste

1 tablespoon olive oil   1/2 teaspoon lemon pepper, plus more to taste

- Rinse salmon fillets with cold water and thoroughly pat dry with paper towels. Brush fillets all over with olive oil and sprinkle with salt and lemon pepper.

- Preheat outdoor grill to high heat, about 500°F.

- Place salmon fillets skin-sides down on grill grate over direct heat. Close grill cover and grill salmon for about 4 minutes. Turn salmon fillets over, close grill cover and continue grilling fillets until internal temperature reaches 130°F, about 4 minutes more.

- Transfer salmon to a serving plate, cover loosely with aluminum foil and let rest for about 5 minutes. Serve 2 fillets immediately as desired. Let remaining 6 fillets cool, cover and refrigerate for later use. Enjoy!

PER SERVING: Calories: 248; Fat: 11g; Protein: 36g; Carbs: 0g; Fiber: 0g Net Carbs: 0g; Fat 42% / Protein 58% / Carbs 0%

Day 1 Dinner: Roasted Chicken

Serves: 2 (plus 2 leftover portions) / Preparation time: 30 minutes / Cooking time: 90 minutes

Cut the carb count on this meal by about 2g per serving by skipping the carrots and serving steamed green beans or broccoli instead.

1 whole roasting chicken (about 4 pounds, giblets removed)

1 tablespoon peanut oil

1 tablespoon mixed dried herbs (such as oregano, thyme and rosemary)

1 teaspoon salt, plus more to taste

1/2 teaspoon freshly ground black pepper, plus more to taste

1 onion (quartered)

2 celery stalks (cut into 2-inch pieces)

4 medium carrots (peeled, quartered)

- Preheat oven to 350°F.

- Rinse chicken with cold water, pat dry with paper towels and brush inside and out with peanut oil. Sprinkle chicken inside and out with herbs, salt and pepper. Place onion and celery in chicken cavity and tie drumsticks together with kitchen twine.

- Place chicken and carrots in roasting pan and roast, uncovered, until internal temperature of chicken reaches 180°F, about 1 1/2 hours.

- Remove roasting pan from oven, cover loosely with foil and let rest for about 10 minutes.

- Cut kitchen twine from drumsticks and remove onion and celery from chicken cavity. Carve breasts from chicken and set aside. Carve remaining chicken, baste with cooking juices and serve immediately with the carrots. Let chicken breasts cool, cover and refrigerate for later use. Enjoy!

PER SERVING: Calories: 277; Fat: 19g; Protein: 22g; Carbs: 6g; Fiber: 2g Net Carbs: 4g; Fat 62% / Protein 32% / Carbs 6%

Day 2 Breakfast: Keto Almond Pancakes

Serves: 4 (plus 2 leftover portions) / Preparation time: 15 minutes / Cooking time: 20 minutes

Toasted almonds add a satisfying crunch to these low-carb pancakes.

- 1/4 cup heavy cream
- 1 1/2 cups almond flour
- 6 tablespoons coconut flour
- 1 tablespoon stevia
- 1 1/2 teaspoons baking powder
- 1/4 teaspoon salt, plus more to taste
- 6 eggs (lightly beaten)
- 1/3 cup unsweetened almond milk
- 3 tablespoons butter (melted)
- 1/2 teaspoon vanilla extract
- Vegetable oil, for greasing skillet
- 1/4 cup sliced almonds (lightly toasted)

- In a small bowl, whip cream with an electric hand mixer until stiff peaks form. Cover bowl and refrigerate until serving.

- In a large bowl, whisk almond flour, coconut flour, stevia, baking powder and salt until thoroughly combined. In a separate bowl, whisk eggs, almond milk, butter and vanilla until thoroughly combined. Make a well in the center of the dry ingredients, pour in egg mixture and whisk until combined (some lumps will remain).

- Heat about 1 teaspoon vegetable oil on a large nonstick griddle over medium heat. Pour batter onto griddle in 1/4 cup portions and cook until surface is bubbly, about 3 minutes. Turn pancakes and cook until lightly browned on the bottom, about 2 minutes. Remove finished pancakes to a serving plate and repeat with remaining batter.

- Divide pancakes in to 3 portions. Top 1 portion of pancakes with whipped cream, sprinkle with almonds and serve immediately. Let remaining 2 portions of pancakes cool, cover and refrigerate for later use. Enjoy!

PER SERVING: Calories: 254; Fat: 24g; Protein: 7g; Carbs: 7g; Fiber: 4g Net Carbs: 3g; Fat 84% / Protein 8% / Carbs 8%

Day 2 Lunch: Pork Medallions

Serves: 4 (plus 2 leftover portions) / Preparation time: 10 minutes / Cooking time: 4 hours

Plan ahead when preparing this recipe--it cooks for 4 hours in a slow cooker. But if you have an Instant Pot, you can cut the cooking time to about 10 minutes! To round out your meal, serve with vinegar-and-oil cole slaw and some fresh seasonal fruit.

- 2 pork tenderloins (about 1 1/2 pounds each)
- 1 tablespoon butter
- 1 teaspoon salt, plus more to taste
- 1/2 teaspoon freshly ground black pepper, plus more to taste
- 1 tablespoon Worcestershire sauce
- 3 garlic cloves (minced)
- 1 onion (sliced)

- Brush pork tenderloins with butter and rub with salt and pepper.

- Place tenderloins in slow cooker, sprinkle with Worcestershire sauce and top with garlic and onions. Cover slow cooker and cook on low setting for 4 hours.

- Remove tenderloins from slow cooker. Cut 1 tenderloin into slices, drizzle with juices from slow cooker and serve immediately. Cut remaining tenderloin in half, let cool, cover and refrigerate for later use. Enjoy!

PER SERVING: Calories: 139; Fat: 4g; Protein: 24g; Carbs: 0g; Fiber: 0g Net Carbs: 0g; Fat 27% / Protein 73% / Carbs 0%

Day 2 Dinner: Mediterranean-Style Salmon

Serves: 2 / Preparation time: 5 minutes / Cooking time: 10 minutes

You can substitute fresh herbs for the dried herb blend. Just wait to add them to the sauce until about 1 minute before serving, or they may become bitter.

1 tablespoon olive oil

2 tablespoons diced onion

1 tomato (diced)

1 teaspoon dried Italian herb blend

Salt and freshly ground black pepper, to taste

2 leftover grilled salmon fillets from Day 1 Lunch

4 ounces feta cheese (crumbled)

6 Kalamata olives (pitted, sliced)

- Heat olive oil in a small saucepan over medium heat and sauté onion until softened, about 5 minutes, stirring occasionally. Add tomato and herbs, season to taste with salt and pepper and heat just to a boil. Reduce heat and simmer until tomatoes are softened, about 5 minutes, stirring occasionally.

- Reheat salmon fillets in the microwave and top with the tomato sauce. Garnish salmon fillets with feta cheese and olives and serve immediately. Enjoy!

PER SERVING: Calories: 345; Fat: 25g; Protein: 25g; Carbs: 6g; Fiber: 1g Net Carbs: 5g; Fat 65% / Protein 29% / Carbs 6%

Day 3 Breakfast: Savory Spinach Crepes

Serves: 4 / Preparation time: 10 minutes / Cooking time: 20 minutes

If you can't find goat cheese or don't especially like it, you could substitute feta cheese (for a similar flavor) or cream cheese (for a milder, less tangy flavor).

- 2 teaspoons extra virgin olive oil (divided)
- 8 ounces (about 6 cups) fresh baby spinach (stems removed)
- 1/4 cup chopped fresh parsley leaves
- 1 tablespoon fresh thyme leaves
- 1 cup (5 ounces) crumbled goat cheese
- 1/2 teaspoon garlic powder
- 1/2 teaspoon onion powder
- 1/4 teaspoon salt
- 1/4 teaspoon freshly ground black pepper
- 1 leftover portion crepes from Day 1 Breakfast
- 1/4 cup (1 ounce) grated Parmesan cheese

- Preheat oven to 350°F. Grease a 9" x 13" casserole dish with 1 teaspoon olive oil and set aside

- Heat remaining 1 teaspoon oil in a large nonstick skillet over medium heat. Add spinach and cover until wilted, about 2 minutes. Add goat cheese, parsley, thyme, garlic powder, onion powder, salt and pepper and stir until cheese is melted.

- Spread mixture up the center of each crepe and roll up to cover filling. Arrange crepes in prepared casserole dish and sprinkle with Parmesan cheese. Cover casserole dish with foil and bake crepes until cheese is melted, about 15 minutes. Serve crepes immediately and enjoy!

PER SERVING: Calories: 300; Fat: 24g; Protein: 19g; Carbs: 4g; Fiber: 1g Net Carbs: 3g; Fat 72% / Protein 25% / Carbs 3%

Day 3 Lunch: Cheeseburger Salad

Serves: 4 (plus 3 leftover portions) / Preparation time: 20 minutes / Cooking time: 15 minutes

Other burger toppings, such as mayonnaise, bacon and onion, would also be tasty in or on these savory salads. Or, turn them into Pizzaburger Salads by using pizza sauce, pizza toppings and cheese instead of the burger ingredients.

3 pounds ground beef

1 tablespoon onion powder

1 tablespoon garlic powder

1 teaspoon salt, plus more to taste

1/2 teaspoon freshly ground black pepper, plus more to taste

1/4 cup sugar-free or reduced-sugar ketchup

2 tablespoons yellow mustard

6 cups torn salad greens

2 dill pickles (sliced)

1 pint (about 2 cups) cherry tomatoes (halved)

1/4 cup (1 ounce) shredded cheddar cheese

- Crumble ground beef in a large nonstick skillet over medium-high heat. Add onion powder, garlic powder, salt and pepper and cook until beef is no longer pink, about 10 minutes, stirring frequently. Drain and discard fat. Remove about 3/4 of the ground beef from the skillet and set aside.

- Add ketchup and mustard to ground beef in skillet and stir until combined.

- Divide salad greens among 4 serving plates. Top greens with ground beef mixture, pickle slices, cherry tomato halves and cheese and serve immediately. Divide reserved ground beef into 3 portions, let cool, cover and refrigerate for later use. Enjoy!

PER SERVING: Calories: 280; Fat: 22g; Protein: 15g; Carbs: 6g; Fiber: 2g Net Carbs: 4g; Fat 71% / Protein 21% / Carbs 8%

Day 3 Dinner: Chicken Taco Bowls

Serves: 4 / Preparation time: 20 minutes / Cooking time: 10 minutes

Diced tomato would be tasty atop these savory taco bowls, and would only add about 3 grams to the net carb count.

1 leftover chicken breast from Day 3 Dinner

1/2 cup salsa

1 teaspoon taco seasoning

1 small head cauliflower (cut into florets)

2 tablespoons butter

1 teaspoon hot sauce

1 teaspoon chili powder

1 teaspoon salt

1 avocado (halved, pitted, sliced)

1/2 cup (2 ounces) shredded cheddar cheese

2 tablespoons sour cream

2 tablespoons sliced black olives

- Shred chicken with a fork, mix with salsa and taco seasoning and heat in the microwave.

- Pulse cauliflower in a food processor until grainy. Melt butter in a large nonstick skillet over medium-high heat and sauté cauliflower until golden, 5 to 6 minutes, stirring frequently. Add hot sauce, chili powder and salt to cauliflower and stir to combine.

- Divide cauliflower among 4 large bowls and top with the chicken mixture. Garnish taco bowls with avocado slices, cheese, sour cream and olives and serve immediately. Enjoy!

PER SERVING: Calories: 350; Fat: 26g; Protein: 22g; Carbs: 9g; Fiber: 5g Net Carbs: 4g; Fat 67% / Protein 25% / Carbs 8%

Day 4 Breakfast: Cinnamon Roll Pancakes

Serves: 4 / Preparation time: 10 minutes

If you have a sweet tooth in the morning, you can add sweetener to the topping mixture before beating.

1 leftover portion pancakes from Day 2 Breakfast

1 package (3 ounces) cream cheese (softened)

1 tablespoon heavy cream

1/4 teaspoon vanilla extract

2 tablespoons butter (softened, divided)

1/2 teaspoon ground cinnamon

1/4 teaspoon ground nutmeg

- Reheat pancakes in the microwave.

- For the topping, in a small bowl, beat cream cheese, heavy cream, vanilla extract and 1 tablespoon butter with an electric hand mixer until slightly fluffy and thoroughly combined. Spread topping over pancakes.

- For the swirl, in a small bowl, mix cinnamon and nutmeg into remaining butter. Drizzle swirl in a spiral pattern over the topping on the pancakes and serve immediately. Enjoy!

**PER SERVING: Calories: 391; Fat: 39g; Protein: 9g; Carbs: 8g; Fiber: 4g
Net Carbs: 4g; Fat 89% / Protein 9% / Carbs 2%**

Day 4 Lunch: Pork "Egg Roll" Bowls

Serves: 4 / Preparation time: 10 minutes / Cooking time: 15 minutes

If your coleslaw mix doesn't have carrots in it, peel and shred one carrot and add it to the wok with the cole slaw mix. It adds a nice dash of color to the finished dish.

2 tablespoons vegetable oil

1 onion (diced)

4 green onions (white and green ends separated, sliced)

4 garlic cloves (minced)

1 bag (14 ounces) coleslaw mix

Salt and freshly ground black pepper, to taste

1 portion leftover pork tenderloin from Day 2 Lunch (shredded)

3 tablespoons soy sauce

1 tablespoon rice wine

1 tablespoon sriracha sauce

1 teaspoon sesame oil

2 tablespoons sesame seeds (toasted)

- Heat oil in a large wok or nonstick skillet over medium-high heat and stir fry onion and the white ends of the green onion until softened, about 5 minutes. Add garlic and stir fry 1 minute more.

- Add coleslaw to wok, season to taste with salt and pepper and stir fry until tender, about 4 minutes. Add shredded pork, soy sauce, rice wine, sriracha and sesame oil and stir until thoroughly combined and heated through.

- Divide pork mixture among 4 large bowls, sprinkle with sesame seeds and green onions and serve immediately. Enjoy!

PER SERVING: Calories: 286; Fat: 15g; Protein: 27g; Carbs: 9g; Fiber: 2g
Net Carbs: 7g; Fat 47% / Protein 38% / Carbs 15%

Day 4 Dinner: Salmon Patties

Serves: 4 / Preparation time: 15 minutes / Cooking time: 10 minutes

Roll up these savory patties in your favorite low-carb sandwich wrap with arugula leaves and aioli.

- 2 leftover grilled salmon fillets from Day 1 Lunch
- 1 egg (lightly beaten)
- 2 tablespoons chopped fresh parsley
- 2 tablespoons Panko breadcrumbs
- 1 tablespoon chopped fresh basil leaves
- 1 lemon (zested, juiced)
- 1 teaspoon onion powder
- Salt, freshly ground black pepper and dried red pepper flakes, to taste
- 1 tablespoon olive oil

- Flake salmon fillets with a fork. Mix salmon, egg, parsley, breadcrumbs, basil, lemon juice and onion powder and season to taste with salt, pepper and red pepper flakes. Stir salmon mixture until thoroughly combined and form into 4 firmly packed patties.

- Heat oil in a large nonstick skillet over medium heat and fry patties until browned on both sides, about 4 minutes per side. Sprinkle patties with lemon zest and serve immediately. Enjoy!

PER SERVING: Calories: 356; Fat: 22g; Protein: 33g; Carbs: 7g; Fiber: 1g Net Carbs: 6g; Fat 56% / Protein 37% / Carbs 7%

Day 5 Breakfast: Bacon Mushroom Crepes

Serves: 4 / Preparation time: 10 minutes / Cooking time: 15 minutes

This is a blurb about the recipe. It says something about the recipe. You could write something about the ingredients, how the food tastes, what the food could be served with, possible substitutions, how healthy it is, or some other information about the recipe. It should be approximately 2 or 3 lines.

4 bacon slices (diced)

8 ounces fresh mushrooms (sliced)

1/4 teaspoon freshly ground black pepper, plus more to taste

1 leftover portion crepes from Day 1 Breakfast

2 tablespoons grated Parmesan cheese

- Fry diced bacon in a medium nonstick skillet over medium heat until browned and crisp, about 8 minutes, stirring frequently. Remove bacon from skillet with a slotted spoon and set aside on paper towels to drain.

- Sauté mushrooms in bacon fat until softened and lightly browned, about 5 minutes, stirring frequently. Drain fat from skillet.

- Reheat crepes in the microwave. Add bacon and pepper to mushrooms and stir to combine. Spoon mushroom mixture up the center of the crepes, roll up and sprinkle with Parmesan cheese to serve. Enjoy!

PER SERVING: Calories: 196; Fat: 15g; Protein: 12g; Carbs: 2g; Fiber: 0g Net Carbs: 2g; Fat 69% / Protein 24% / Carbs 7%

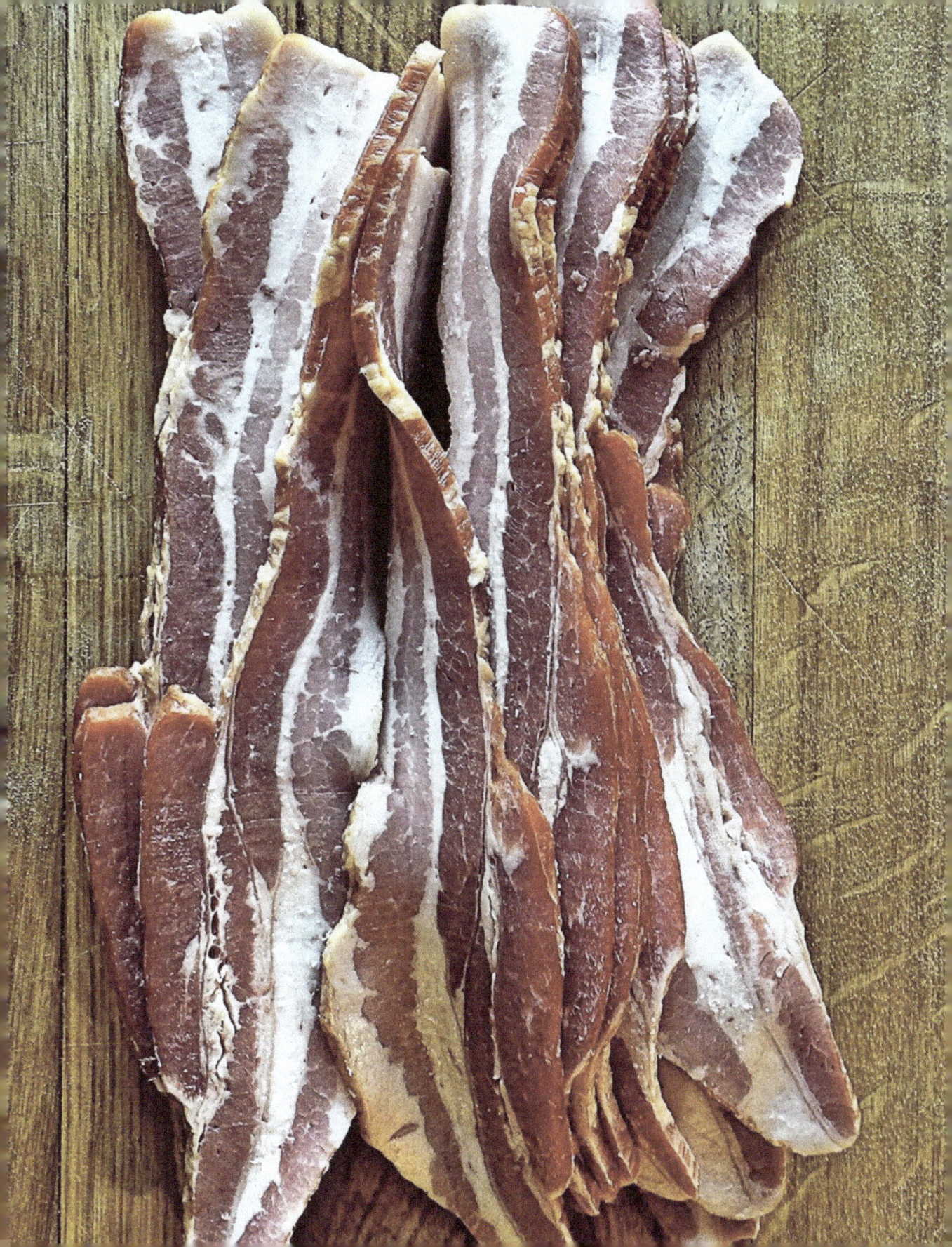

Day 5 Lunch: Stuffed Green Peppers

Serves: 4 / Preparation time: 15 minutes / Cooking time: 30 minutes

Green bell peppers are the lowest-carb bell peppers. You could substitute tomatoes for the peppers without affecting your carb count. Using red or yellow bell peppers will increase the carb count by 1 and 2 grams respectively.

1 leftover portion ground beef from Day 3 Lunch

2 eggs (lightly beaten)

1 tablespoon dried Italian herb blend

Salt and freshly ground black pepper, to taste

1/2 cup (2 ounces) shredded mozzarella cheese (divided)

2 tablespoons (1/2 ounce) grated Parmesan cheese (divided)

4 green bell peppers

- Preheat oven to 350°F. Spray a glass 8" x 8" baking pan with nonstick cooking spray.
- Cut tops from peppers and remove seeds and ribs, leaving peppers intact.
- In a large bowl, mix ground beef, eggs, herbs and about half of the cheeses until thoroughly combined. Stuff meat mixture into peppers.
- Arrange peppers in prepared baking pan, top with remaining cheeses and bake until cheese is melted and peppers are tender, about 30 minutes. Serve immediately and enjoy!

PER SERVING: Calories: 337; Fat: 23g; Protein: 24g; Carbs: 9g; Fiber: 2g Net Carbs: 7g; Fat 61% / Protein 28% / Carbs 11%

Day 5 Dinner: Chicken Tikka Masala

Serves: 3 / Preparation time: 10 minutes / Cooking time: 15 minutes

Serve this saucy Indian-style chicken with naan or roti (Indian flatbreads) or cauliflower rice.

- 1 tablespoon butter
- 2 tablespoons chopped onion
- 2 garlic cloves (minced)
- 1 teaspoon turmeric
- 1/2 teaspoon ground ginger
- 1/4 teaspoon ground coriander
- 1/4 teaspoon ground cumin
- 1/4 teaspoon chili powder
- 1/4 teaspoon salt, plus more to taste
- Pinch cinnamon
- Freshly ground black pepper, to taste
- 1/2 cup heavy cream
- 1/4 cup sour cream
- 1 tablespoon tomato paste
- 1 leftover chicken breast from Day 3 Dinner (cut into bite-size pieces)
- Chopped fresh cilantro leaves, for garnish

- Melt butter in a medium nonstick skillet over medium heat and sauté onion until translucent, stirring frequently, about 5 minutes. Add garlic and sauté about 1 minute more, stirring constantly. Add spices and stir until onions and garlic are coated and spices are fragrant.

- Add heavy cream, sour cream and tomato paste to skillet and stir until thoroughly combined. Add chicken and stir until coated.

- Reduce heat to medium-low, cover skillet and simmer for about 5 minutes. Remove cover and simmer to reduce sauce to desired consistency. Season tikka masala to taste with salt and pepper, garnish with cilantro leaves and serve immediately. Enjoy!

PER SERVING: Calories: 280; Fat: 23g; Protein: 15g; Carbs: 3g; Fiber: 0g Net Carbs: 3g; Fat 74% / Protein 21% / Carbs 5%

Day 6 Breakfast: Raspberry Pancakes

Serves: 4 (plus 1 leftover portion) / Preparation time: 5 minutes / Cooking time: 15 minutes

Raspberries and blackberries are the lowest-carb berries, at 5 grams of net carbs per serving. Strawberries come in a close second at 6 grams of net carbs per serving. So any of those berries, or a mixture of them, could be used in this recipe with little impact on the net carb count.

1 pint (12 ounces) fresh or frozen raspberries

1 cup water, plus more as needed

Sweetener of choice equivalent to 1 tablespoon sugar

1 lemon (zested, juiced)

1/4 teaspoon ground ginger

1 teaspoon cornstarch

1 leftover portion pancakes from Day 2 Breakfast

- In small saucepan over medium heat, mix raspberries, water, sweetener, lemon juice and ginger and heat just to a simmer, stirring frequently. Reduce heat and simmer for about 10 minutes, stirring occasionally.

- Mix cornstarch with about 1 tablespoon cold water, stir into raspberry mixture and simmer until thickened, stirring constantly, about 1 minute. Divide sauce into 2 portions.

- Reheat pancakes in the microwave, drizzle with 1 portion of the sauce and sprinkle with lemon zest to serve. Let remaining portion of sauce cool, cover and refrigerate for later use. Enjoy!

PER SERVING: Calories: 276; Fat: 24g; Protein: 7g; Carbs: 12g; Fiber: 7g Net Carbs: 5g; Fat 78% / Protein 10% / Carbs 12%

Day 6 Lunch: Spinach and Salmon Salad with Strawberry Vinaigrette

Serves: 4 / Preparation time: 10 minutes

Any salad greens can be used for this recipe, but the combination of fresh spinach and fresh strawberries is hard to beat!

1 bag (10 ounces) fresh baby spinach leaves

2 leftover grilled salmon fillets from Day 1 Lunch (coarsely flaked)

2 tablespoons fresh basil

2 cups fresh strawberry halves (divided)

3 tablespoons balsamic vinegar

1 small knob (about 1/2") fresh ginger

1 teaspoon honey

1/4 cup chopped pecans (toasted)

- In a large bowl, toss spinach, salmon, basil and 1 1/2 cups of the strawberries.

- For the dressing, pulse remaining 1/2 cup strawberries with the vinegar, ginger and honey. until smooth. Drizzle dressing over salad, sprinkle with pecans and serve immediately. Enjoy!

PER SERVING: Calories: 139; Fat: 7g; Protein: 11g; Carbs: 10g; Fiber: 3g Net Carbs: 7g; Fat 45% / Protein 32% / Carbs 23%

Day 6 Dinner: Slow Cooker Pulled Ham

Serves: 2 (plus 4 leftover portions) / Preparation time: 20 minutes / Cooking time: 6 to 8 hours

Vinegar-and-oil cole slaw and fresh seasonal steamed vegetables would perfectly complement this tender, savory ham.

1 fully cooked bone-in shank or butt portion half ham (about 4 pounds)

1 cup cider vinegar

1/4 cup packed brown sugar

1 tablespoon Worcestershire sauce

1 teaspoon red pepper flakes

1/2 teaspoon freshly ground black pepper, plus more to taste

- Place ham cut-side down in slow cooker (cut ham into chunks if necessary for fit).

- In a small bowl, whisk vinegar, brown sugar, Worcestershire sauce, red pepper flakes and pepper until thoroughly combined and pour over ham.

- Cover slow cooker and cook on low setting until ham is very tender, 6 to 8 hours.

- Remove ham from slow cooker and shred with two forks, leaving some meat on the bone. Divide meat into 5 portions and serve one portion immediately as desired. Let bone and remaining 4 portions cool, cover and refrigerate for later use. Enjoy!

PER SERVING: Calories: 130; Fat: 7g; Protein: 14g; Carbs: 6g; Fiber: 0g Net Carbs: 6g; Fat 48% / Protein 43% / Carbs 9%

Day 7 Breakfast: Egg and Sausage Bake

Serves: 4 (plus 2 leftover portions) / Preparation time: 20 minutes / Cooking time: 40 minutes

For extra taste, you can add crushed fennel seeds and red pepper flakes to the sausage mixture. Or, to ease preparation, use breakfast sausage that's already seasoned.

- 1 teaspoon vegetable oil
- 12 ounces ground pork
- 1 small white onion (diced)
- 2 garlic cloves (minced)
- 1 teaspoon ground sage
- 1 teaspoon dried thyme
- 1/2 teaspoon salt, plus more to taste
- 1/4 teaspoon freshly ground black pepper, plus more to taste
- 12 eggs (beaten)
- 1/4 cup sour cream
- 1/4 cup heavy cream
- 2 cups (8 ounces) shredded mild cheddar cheese (divided)

- Preheat oven to 350°F. Grease a glass 9" x 13" casserole dish with vegetable oil and set aside.

- Crumble sausage in a large nonstick skillet over medium heat. Add onion, garlic, sage and thyme, garlic, salt and pepper and cook until sausage is browned, stirring frequently, about 10 minutes. Drain fat from sausage if necessary, add salt and pepper and stir until combined.

- Spread sausage mixture in prepared casserole dish and set aside.

- Whisk eggs, sour cream and heavy cream. Add about half of the cheese, season to taste with salt and pepper and stir to combine. Pour egg mixture over sausage in casserole dish and top with about half of the cheese.

- Bake casserole until eggs are set and top is lightly browned, about 30 minutes. Divide casserole into 3 portions. Sprinkle cheese over 1 portion and serve immediately. Let remaining 2 portions of casserole cool, cover and refrigerate for later use. Enjoy!

PER SERVING: Calories: 251; Fat: 20g; Protein: 16g; Carbs: 2g; Fiber: 0g Net Carbs: 2g; Fat 72% / Protein 25% / Carbs 3%

Day 7 Lunch: Beef with Zoodles

Serves: 4 / Preparation time: 15 minutes / Cooking time: 10 minutes

If you don't have a spiralizer, you could use a vegetable peeler to make the zoodles, or cut them into thin matchstick strips.

- 2 tablespoons butter
- 4 medium zucchini (about 8 ounces each)(spiralized)
- 1 teaspoon sesame oil
- 1 teaspoon garlic powder
- 1 teaspoon onion powder
- 1/2 teaspoon ground ginger
- Salt and freshly ground black pepper, to taste
- 1 leftover portion ground beef from Day 3 Lunch
- 1 tablespoon soy sauce
- 1 teaspoon sriracha sauce
- 1 teaspoon sesame seeds (toasted)

- Melt butter in a large nonstick skillet over medium heat. Add zucchini, sesame oil, garlic powder, onion powder and ginger, season to taste with salt and pepper and stir fry until soft and lightly golden, about 6 minutes.

- Crumble ground beef, add to zucchini mixture with soy sauce and sriracha sauce and stir until heated through. Transfer to a serving bowl and sprinkle with sesame seeds to serve. Enjoy!

PER SERVING: Calories: 295; Fat: 25g; Protein: 16g; Carbs: 1g; Fiber: 3g Net Carbs: 3g; Fat 76% / Protein 22% / Carbs 2%

Day 7 Dinner: Cashew Pork Stir Fry

Serves: 4 / Preparation time: 15 minutes / Cooking time: 15 minutes

This recipe calls for roasted, salted cashew halves. You could use unsalted nuts, but you may need to increase the soy sauce or add some salt to the dish.

- 2 tablespoons vegetable oil
- 1 red bell pepper (sliced)
- 2 green onions (white and green ends separated, sliced)
- 2 garlic cloves (minced)
- 1 teaspoon sesame oil
- 2 eggs (lightly beaten)
- 2 tablespoons soy sauce
- 1 teaspoon ground ginger
- Freshly ground black pepper, to taste
- 1 portion leftover pork tenderloin from Day 2 Lunch (cut into thin 1" strips)
- 1/2 cup dry roasted salted cashew halves

- Heat vegetable oil in a wok or large nonstick skillet over medium-high heat and stir fry bell pepper and white ends of green onions until softened, about 5 minutes. Add garlic and sesame oil and stir fry about 1 minute more.

- Whisk egg, soy sauce and ginger, season to taste with pepper, add to wok and stir fry until egg is cooked through, about 4 minutes.

- Add pork and cashews to wok and stir until heated through. Sprinkle stir fry with green onions, serve immediately and enjoy!

PER SERVING: Calories: 323; Fat: 20g; Protein: 28g; Carbs: 9g; Fiber: 2g Net Carbs: 7g; Fat 56% / Protein 35% / Carbs 8%

Day 8 Breakfast: Raspberry Cheesecake Smoothies

Serves: 2 / Preparation time: 5 minutes

Adding a cup of fresh or frozen strawberries, raspberries or blackberries to this smoothie recipe would increase the net carbs of each serving by just 2 grams.

3 cups unsweetened almond milk

12 to 15 ice cubes

1 leftover portion raspberry sauce from Day 6 Breakfast

1 package (3 ounces) cream cheese (softened)

1/4 teaspoon vanilla extract

- Place all ingredients in a blender container and pulse until smooth. Serve immediately and enjoy!

PER SERVING: Calories: 202; Fat: 18g; Protein: 4g; Carbs: 8g; Fiber: 2g Net Carbs: 6g; Fat 80% / Protein 8% / Carbs 12%

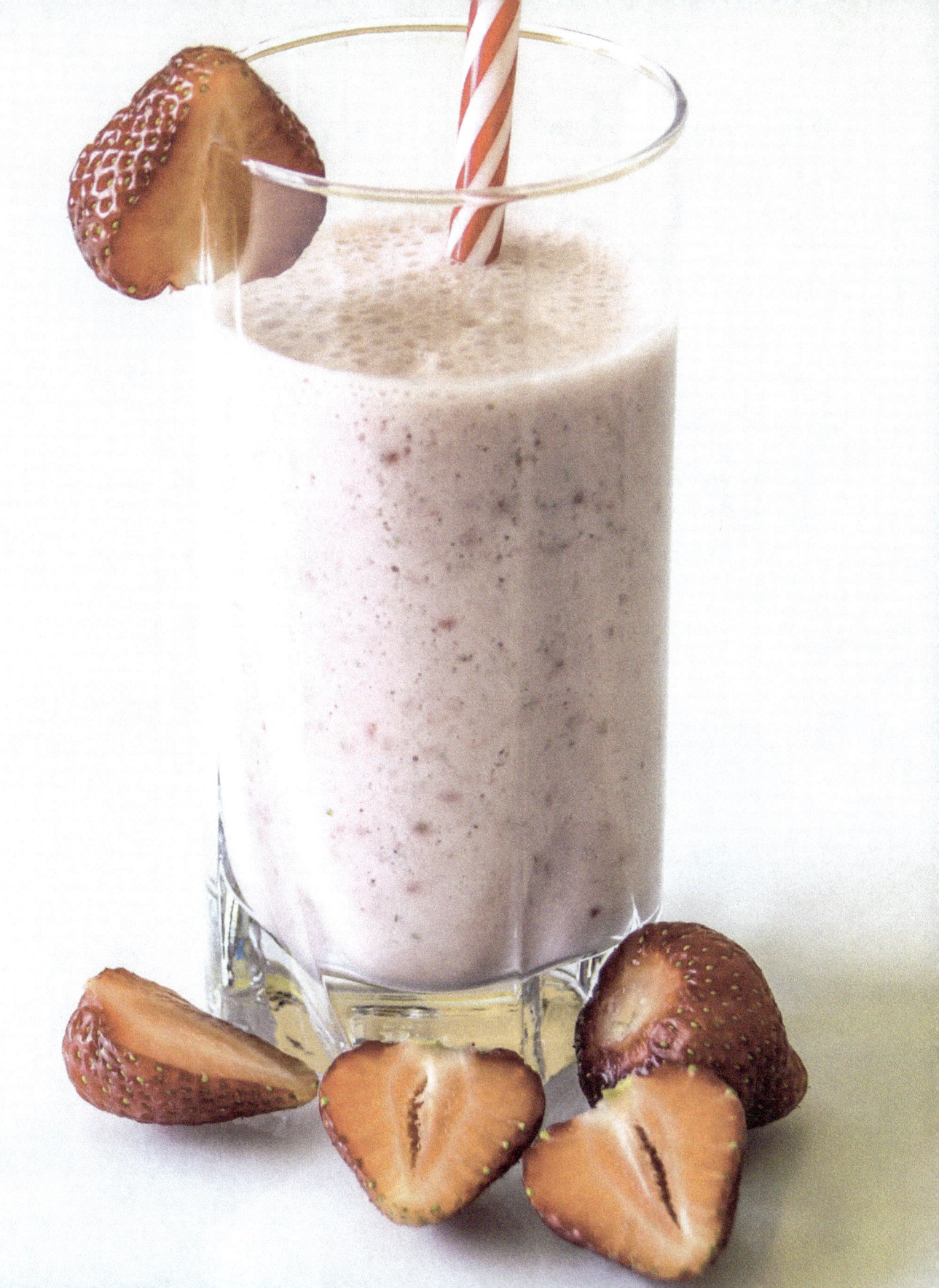

Day 8 Lunch: Ham Roll-Ups

Serves: 2 / Preparation time: 15 minutes

Feel free to substitute your favorite low-carb sandwich wraps for the lettuce leaves, if you can spare the carbs.

- 1 tablespoon cream cheese (softened)
- 1 tablespoon mayonnaise
- 1 teaspoon Dijon mustard
- 1/4 teaspoon freshly ground black pepper
- 4 large lettuce leaves
- 1 leftover portion pulled ham from Day 6 Dinner
- 1/4 cup diced red bell pepper
- 1 dill pickle (sliced)

- For the dressing, in a small bowl, mix cream cheese, mayonnaise, mustard and black pepper until thoroughly combined.

- Layer pairs of lettuce leaves together. Spread half of the dressing up the center of each pair of leaves and top with ham, bell pepper and pickle slices.

- Tightly roll lettuce leaves around filling and secure with decorative toothpicks, if desired. Serve roll-ups immediately and enjoy!

PER SERVING: Calories: 219; Fat: 15g; Protein: 16g; Carbs: 9g; Fiber: 2g Net Carbs: 7g; Fat 62% / Protein 29% / Carbs 8%

Day 8 Dinner: Chicken Breasts with Lemon Dill Butter

Serves: 2 (plus 2 leftover portions) / Preparation time: 15 minutes / Cooking time: 25 minutes

You can use dried dill in this recipe instead of fresh, but reduce the amount to about 1 teaspoon.

- 2 tablespoons butter (softened)
- 1 tablespoon chopped fresh dill
- 1 teaspoon lemon juice
- 1/2 teaspoon garlic powder
- 2 tablespoons olive oil
- 6 boneless skinless chicken breasts
- 1/2 teaspoon salt, plus more to taste
- 1/4 teaspoon freshly ground black pepper, plus more to taste
- 2 tablespoons olive oil

- For the lemon dill butter, in a small bowl, mix butter, dill, lemon juice and garlic powder until thoroughly combined and refrigerate until serving.

- Sprinkle chicken breasts all over with salt and pepper.

- Heat olive oil in a large nonstick skillet over medium-high heat and sear chicken breasts until lightly browned on both sides. Reduce heat and cook chicken until internal temperature reaches 165°F, about 20 minutes, turning as necessary.

- Cut 2 chicken breasts into slices and serve with the herb butter. Let remaining chicken breasts cool, cover and refrigerate for later use. Enjoy!

PER SERVING: Calories: 362; Fat: 29g; Protein: 25g; Carbs: 0g; Fiber: 0g Net Carbs: 0g; Fat 72% / Protein 28% / Carbs 0%

Day 9 Breakfast: Zucchini and Onion Eggs

Serves: 4 / Preparation time: 10 minutes / Cooking time: 10 minutes

If you're using a portion of a larger zucchini instead of a whole medium-sized one, you may want to remove the seeds before shredding.

1 tablespoon butter

1 medium white onion (sliced)

1 medium zucchini (shredded)

Salt and freshly ground black pepper, to taste

1 leftover portion egg and sausage bake from Day 7 Breakfast

- Melt butter in a medium nonstick skillet and sauté onion and zucchini until softened and lightly golden, about 6 minutes, stirring occasionally. Season zucchini mixture to taste with salt and pepper.

- Reheat egg and sausage bake in the microwave and crumble into a serving dish. Top with zucchini mixture and serve immediately. Enjoy!

PER SERVING: Calories: 170; Fat: 14g; Protein: 9g; Carbs: 4g; Fiber: 0g Net Carbs: 4g; Fat 74% / Protein 21% / Carbs 5%

Day 9 Lunch: Broccoli Beef Alfredo

Serves: 4 / Preparation time: 15 minutes / Cooking time: 15 minutes

To further reduce your carb intake, you could prepare this dish with mushrooms instead of the broccoli. To do this, sauté 2 cups of sliced fresh mushrooms in the butter for about 5 minutes before proceeding with the recipe as written.

1 package (10 ounces) frozen broccoli florets

2 tablespoons butter (melted)

1/2 cup heavy cream

1/2 cup (2 ounces) grated Parmesan cheese

1 teaspoon garlic powder

1 teaspoon onion powder

1 teaspoon Italian herb blend, plus more for garnish

1 leftover portion ground beef from Day 3 Lunch

1/4 cup (1 ounce) shredded mozzarella cheese

- Steam broccoli according to the package directions.

- For the sauce, melt butter in a medium saucepan over medium heat. Add cream, Parmesan cheese, garlic powder, onion powder and herb blend, season to taste with salt and pepper and whisk until sauce is smooth and cheese is melted.

- Add broccoli and beef to sauce and stir until thoroughly combined. Transfer broccoli beef Alfredo to a serving bowl, sprinkle with mozzarella cheese and garnish with additional herb blend to serve. Enjoy!

PER SERVING: Calories: 481; Fat: 40g; Protein: 26g; Carbs: 5g; Fiber: 2g Net Carbs: 3g; Fat 75% / Protein 22% / Carbs 3%

Day 9 Dinner: Chicken Cordon Bleu Casserole

Serves: 8 / Preparation time: 15 minutes / Cooking time: 40 minutes

If you have any leftovers of this meaty, cheesy and creamy casserole, you could use it as a decadent filling for quesadillas!

2 leftover chicken breasts from Day 8 Dinner (shredded)

1 leftover portion pulled ham from Day 6 Dinner

4 tablespoons butter

6 ounces cream cheese

2 tablespoons lemon juice

1 tablespoon Dijon mustard

1/2 tablespoon freshly ground black pepper, plus more to taste

6 slices (1 ounce each) Swiss cheese

- Preheat oven to 350°F. Spray a glass 9" x 13" baking dish with nonstick cooking spray.
- Spread shredded chicken in prepared baking dish and top with pulled ham.
- For the sauce, melt butter in a small saucepan. Add cream cheese, lemon juice, mustard and pepper to pan and stir until sauce is smooth and thoroughly combined.
- Evenly pour sauce over chicken and ham and top with cheese slices.
- Bake casserole until heated through and cheese is melted and lightly browned, 30 to 35 minutes.
- Let casserole stand for about 5 minutes before serving. Enjoy!

PER SERVING: Calories: 348; Fat: 26g; Protein: 24g; Carbs: 2g; Fiber: 0g Net Carbs: 2g; Fat 67% / Protein 28% / Carbs 5%

Day 10 Breakfast: Bacon Cheddar Scramble

Serves: 2 (plus 3 leftover portions) / Preparation time: 10 minutes / Cooking time: 15 minutes

For a more intense cheese flavor, use sharp cheddar cheese instead of the mild. If cheddar isn't to your taste, you could use feta or Monterey Jack cheese instead.

1 package (16 ounces) bacon (cut into 1/2" cubes)

4 eggs (beaten)

1/4 cup (1 ounce) shredded mild cheddar cheese

2 tablespoons half-and-half

1/4 teaspoon onion powder

1/4 teaspoon garlic powder

Salt and freshly ground black pepper, to taste

- Sauté bacon in a large nonstick skillet over medium heat until browned, stirring frequently, about 10 minutes. Remove bacon from skillet with a slotted spoon and drain on paper towels. Pour bacon drippings into a heatproof container, discarding solids, and set aside.

- In a medium bowl, whisk eggs, cheese, half-and-half, onion powder and garlic powder until thoroughly combined and season to taste with salt and pepper.

- Heat 1 tablespoon bacon drippings in skillet, add egg mixture and cook over medium heat, stirring frequently, until eggs are cooked through and nearly set, about 5 minutes.

- Divide bacon into 4 portions. Sprinkle 1 portion bacon over eggs, stir until heated through and serve immediately. Let remaining 3 portions of bacon cool, cover and refrigerate for later use. Let remaining bacon drippings cool, divide into 3 portions, cover and refrigerate for later use. Enjoy!

PER SERVING: Calories: 267; Fat: 20g; Protein: 20g; Carbs: 2g; Fiber: 0g Net Carbs: 2g; Fat 67% / Protein 30% / Carbs 3%

Day 10 Lunch: Ham and Cheddar Crepes

Serves: 4 / Preparation time: 5 minutes / Cooking time: 20 minutes

For extra savory flavor, add some onion powder and/or garlic powder to the egg mixture before frying the crepes.

- 4 eggs (lightly beaten)
- 1/4 cup heavy cream
- Freshly ground black pepper, to taste
- 4 teaspoons butter (divided)
- 1 leftover portion pulled ham from Day 6 Dinner
- 1/2 cup (2 ounces) shredded cheddar cheese
- 2 tablespoons fresh chopped chives

- In a large bowl, whisk eggs and cream and season to taste with pepper. Melt 1 teaspoon butter in a medium nonstick skillet over medium heat. Pour about 1/4 of the egg mixture into pan, swirl pan to coat evenly and let cook for about 2 minutes.

- Sprinkle about 1/4 of the ham and 1/4 of the cheese over egg in pan and cook until cheese is melted, about 2 minutes more. Roll up crepe over filling, remove from pan and set aside. Repeat with remaining eggs, ham and cheese.

- Sprinkle chives over crepes, serve and enjoy!

PER SERVING: Calories: 345; Fat: 26g; Protein: 24g; Carbs: 7g; Fiber: 0g Net Carbs: 7g; Fat 68% / Protein 28% / Carbs 4%

Day 10 Dinner: Grilled Burgers

Serves: 4 (plus 2 leftover portions) / Preparation time: 30 minutes / Cooking time: 10 minutes

Be sure to use keto-friendly mayonnaise when you're on a keto diet. Look for high-quality mayonnaise that's low in sugar and made with a high-quality oil, like avocado oil.

3 pounds fresh ground chuck

4 slices raw bacon (minced)

4 eggs (lightly beaten)

1/4 cup mayonnaise, plus more for serving

1/4 cup sriracha sauce

1 tablespoon onion powder

1 tablespoon onion powder

1 tablespoon salt

1 tablespoon crushed red pepper flakes

1 1/2 teaspoons freshly ground black pepper

Green leaf lettuce

4 slices (1 ounce each) American cheese

1 large tomato (sliced)

- In a large bowl, mix ground chuck, bacon, eggs, mayonnaise, sriracha sauce, onion powder, garlic powder, salt, red pepper flakes and pepper just until combined (do not over mix). Divide meat mixture into 12 portions and form into patties.

- Preheat grill to high heat.

- Place patties on grill grate and cook to desired doneness, about 5 minutes per side (burgers should cook until internal temperature reaches at least 140°F).

- Place large lettuce leaves on 4 plates. Top each with a burger, a slice of cheese, tomato slices and dollops of mayonnaise and serve immediately. Let remaining 8 burgers cool, cover and refrigerate for later use. Enjoy!

PER SERVING: Calories: 440; Fat: 34g; Protein: 28g; Carbs: 5g; Fiber: 1g Net Carbs: 4g; Fat 70% / Protein 25% / Carbs 5%

Day 11 Breakfast: Tzatziki Eggs

Serves: 4 / Preparation time: 10 minutes

If you can't find Kalamata olives, you could use large black olives. Note that Kalamata olives are milder and less salty than black olives, so keep this in mind when seasoning the sauce with salt.

- 1 small cucumber (seeded, chopped)
- 1/4 cup sour cream
- 1/2 teaspoon dried dill
- Salt and freshly ground black pepper, to taste
- 1 leftover portion egg and sausage bake from Day 7 Breakfast
- 1 tomato (seeded, diced)
- 1/2 cup sliced pitted Kalamata olives

- For the tzatziki sauce, mix cucumber, sour cream and dill, season to taste with salt and pepper and set aside.
- Reheat egg and sausage bake in the microwave, sprinkle with tomato and olives and top with tzatziki sauce. Serve immediately and enjoy!

PER SERVING: Calories: 219; Fat: 18g; Protein: 10g; Carbs: 7g; Fiber: 1g
Net Carbs: 6g; Fat 74% / Protein 18% / Carbs 8%

Day 11 Lunch: Egg Bites with Bacon

Serves: 4 (plus 9 leftover hard boiled eggs) / Preparation time: 45 minutes / Cooking time: 20 minutes

Change the look of these savory bites by mixing the bacon into the egg mixture and rolling the balls in the shredded cheese.

12 eggs

6 bacon slices

1 package (3 ounces) cream cheese (softened)

1/4 cup shredded sharp cheddar cheese

3 tablespoons butter (softened)

1 tablespoon mayonnaise

1 teaspoon dried dill

Freshly ground black pepper, to taste

- Fill a large saucepan half-full with water and heat to a boil. Gently lower eggs into water with a kitchen tongs or small mesh strainer. Reduce heat to a simmer and cook eggs for 13 minutes. Remove eggs from the boiling water, submerge in an ice water bath and let cool for about 5 minutes. Peel eggs and set aside.

- While the eggs are cooking, fry bacon in a large nonstick skillet until crispy. Remove bacon from skillet and set aside on paper towels, reserving bacon fat.

- Mash 3 peeled eggs in a medium bowl with cream cheese, cheddar cheese, butter, mayonnaise, dill and reserved bacon fat and season to taste with pepper. Cover bowl and refrigerate until chilled through, about 30 minutes. Place remaining 9 eggs in a covered container and refrigerate for later use.

- Mince cooked bacon. Divide chilled egg mixture into 8 portions and form into balls. Roll each ball in minced bacon to coat, serve immediately and enjoy!

PER SERVING: Calories: 362; Fat: 34g; Protein: 12g; Carbs: 2g; Fiber: 1g Net Carbs: 1g; Fat 85% / Protein 14% / Carbs 1%

Day 11 Dinner: Pesto Chicken

Serves: 4 / Preparation time: 15 minutes / Cooking time: 20 minutes

For a milder pesto, use spinach leaves in place of some or all of the basil leaves. You could also substitute walnuts for the pine nuts, and/or use Parmesan cheese instead of the Romano.

1/4 cup pine nuts

1 cup fresh basil leaves (stems removed)

2 garlic cloves (minced)

1 teaspoon lemon juice

1/4 teaspoon salt, plus more to taste

1/4 cup extra virgin olive oil

1/4 cup grated Romano cheese

1 tablespoon butter

2 leftover chicken breasts from Day 8 Dinner (cut into 1/4" slices)

Freshly ground black pepper, to taste

- For the pesto, toast pine nuts In a dry skillet over medium heat until lightly browned, stirring frequently, 2 to 3 minutes. Pulse pine nuts, basil leaves, garlic, lemon juice and salt in a food processor until finely minced. While processing, add oil in a slow, thin stream and continue processing until smooth. Add Romano cheese and process just until combined.

- Melt butter in a large nonstick skillet over medium heat. Season chicken slices to taste with salt and pepper and fry in butter until lightly browned on both sides, about 4 minutes. Arrange chicken slices on a large platter and drizzle with pesto to serve. Enjoy!

PER SERVING: Calories: 288; Fat: 24g; Protein: 14g; Carbs: 4g; Fiber: 0g Net Carbs: 4g; Fat 75% / Protein 19% / Carbs 6%

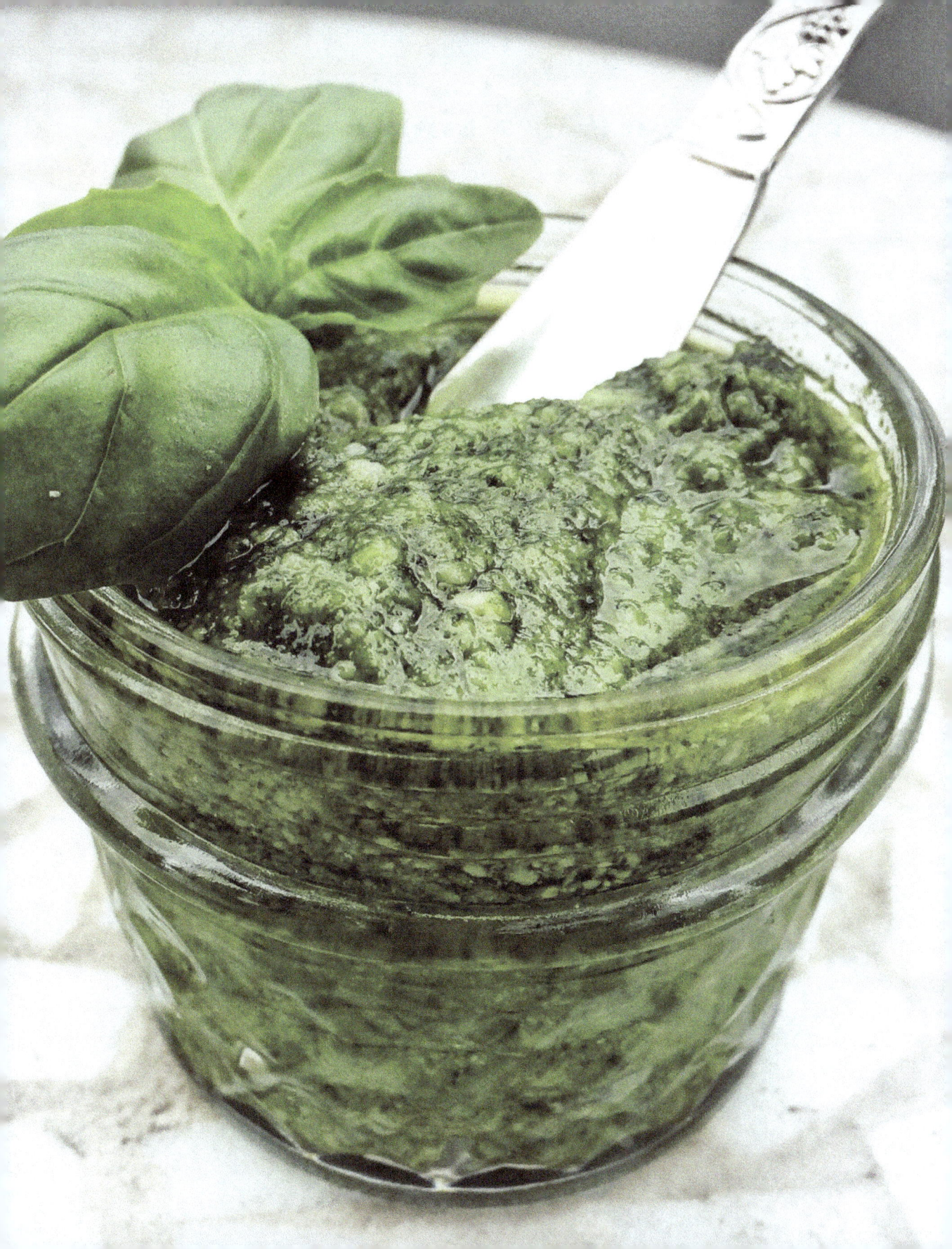

Day 12 Breakfast: Ham & Swiss Frittata

Serves: 4 / Preparation time: 20 minutes / Cooking time: 40 minutes

For a dash of color, you could sprinkle some sliced chives into the egg mixture or over the frittata. Using 2 tablespoons will only negligently affect your carb count.

1 tablespoon butter

1 small onion (sliced)

6 eggs

2 tablespoons heavy cream

1 tablespoon honey mustard

1/4 teaspoon freshly ground black pepper, plus more to taste

1 leftover portion pulled ham from Day 6 Dinner

1 cup (4 ounces) shredded Swiss cheese

- Preheat oven to 350°F. Spray a 9" glass pie pan with nonstick cooking spray.

- Melt butter in a small nonstick skillet and sauté onions until caramelized, stirring occasionally, about 8 minutes.

- In a large bowl, whisk eggs, cream, honey mustard and pepper until thoroughly combined. Add caramelized onion, ham and about half of the cheese and stir until combined. Pour egg mixture into prepared pie pan and sprinkle with remaining cheese.

- Bake frittata until eggs are cooked through and cheese is melted and lightly browned, about 30 minutes. Let frittata stand for about 10 minutes before cutting into wedges to serve. Enjoy!

PER SERVING: Calories: 317; Fat: 21g; Protein: 26g; Carbs: 9g; Fiber: 2g Net Carbs: 7g; Fat 60% / Protein 33% / Carbs 7%

Day 12 Lunch: Wilted Spinach Salad

Serves: 4 (plus 2 leftover portions) / Preparation time: 15 minutes / Cooking time: 20 minutes

Keep a close eye on the spinach after adding it to the skillet so it doesn't wilt too much or too little, according to your own personal preference.

- 12 eggs
- 1 leftover portion bacon drippings from Day 10 Breakfast
- 1 small red onion (thinly sliced)
- 1/4 cup white vinegar
- 2 tablespoons water
- 1 tablespoon sugar
- 1/2 teaspoon salt, plus more to taste
- 1/4 teaspoon freshly ground black pepper, plus more to taste
- 1 bag (10 ounces) fresh baby spinach leaves
- 1 leftover portion bacon from Day 10 Breakfast

- Fill a large saucepan half-full with water and heat to a boil. Gently lower eggs into boiling water with a kitchen tongs and let water return to a boil. Reduce heat to a simmer and cook eggs for 13 minutes. Remove eggs from boiling water and immediately submerge in an ice water bath. Let eggs cool for 5 minutes, peel and set aside.

- Heat bacon drippings in a large nonstick skillet over medium heat and sauté onion until softened, about 4 minutes, stirring occasionally. Add vinegar, water, sugar, salt and pepper and heat to a boil. Remove skillet from heat, add spinach leaves and toss to coat.

- Coarsely chop 4 hard boiled eggs, add to spinach mixture with bacon and toss to coat. Transfer salad to a serving bowl and serve immediately. Cover remaining hard boiled eggs and refrigerate for later use. Enjoy!

PER SERVING: Calories: 164; Fat: 10g; Protein: 10g; Carbs: 8g; Fiber: 2g Net Carbs: 6g; Fat 55% / Protein 25% / Carbs 20%

Day 12 Dinner: Pizza Burgers

Serves: 4 / Preparation time: 20 minutes / Cooking time: 20 minutes

If the cheese on these pizza burgers isn't browned to your taste by the time the burgers are heated through, you could broil them for a few minutes. But watch them closely, so they don't burn!

4 leftover burgers from Day 10 Dinner

16 pepperoni slices

1/4 cup pizza sauce

1/4 cup (1 ounce) grated Parmesan cheese

1 Roma tomato (sliced)

4 slices (1 ounce each) mozzarella cheese

Fresh basil, for garnish

- Preheat oven to 375°F. Spray a rimmed baking sheet with nonstick cooking spray.

- Arrange burgers on prepared baking sheet and top with pepperoni, pizza sauce, Parmesan cheese, tomato slices and mozzarella cheese. Bake pizza burgers until heated through and cheese is melted and lightly browned, about 20 minutes.

- Garnish pizza burgers with fresh basil as desired and serve immediately. Enjoy!

PER SERVING: Calories: 390; Fat: 26g; Protein: 33g; Carbs: 4g; Fiber: 1g Net Carbs: 3g; Fat 60% / Protein 34% / Carbs 6%

Day 13 Breakfast: Brunch Meat Loaf

Serves: 4 (plus 2 leftover portions) / Preparation time: 10 minutes / Cooking time: 70 minutes

For an early-morning serving time, prepare the meat mixture the day before, wrap loaves in foil and refrigerate. On serving day, unwrap loaves, place in baking pan and place the pan in the oven during oven preheating time. The loaves may take a few extra minutes to finish cooking.

- 2 pounds ground pork
- 2 eggs (lightly beaten)
- 1 tablespoon chopped fresh sage
- 1 tablespoon chopped fresh thyme
- 2 teaspoons salt, plus more to taste
- 1 teaspoon onion powder
- 1 teaspoon garlic powder
- 1 teaspoon fennel seeds (crushed)
- 1/2 teaspoon freshly ground black pepper, plus more to taste
- 1/2 teaspoon smoked paprika
- 1/2 teaspoon dried red pepper flakes (crushed)

- Preheat oven to 350°F.
- In a large bowl, mix all ingredients until thoroughly combined. Divide mixture into 3 portions and form each portion into a loaf shape.
- Place meat loaves in an ungreased 13 x 9 inch baking pan. Bake until internal temperature of meat loaves reaches 160°F, 60 to 70 minutes.
- Cut one meat loaf into slices and serve immediately. Let remaining 2 loaves cool, wrap in aluminum foil and refrigerate for later use. Enjoy!

PER SERVING: Calories: 167; Fat: 12g; Protein: 15g; Carbs: 0g; Fiber: 0g Net Carbs: 0g; Fat 65% / Protein 35% / Carbs 0%

Day 13 Lunch: Tuna Salad

Serves: 4 / Preparation time: 20 minutes

Store portions of this tuna salad in jars for quick and easy lunches on-the-go!

1/2 cup cottage cheese

1/2 cup sour cream

1 tablespoon heavy cream (plus more if needed)

2 tablespoons diced red bell pepper

1 1/2 teaspoons minced fresh chives

Salt and freshly ground black pepper, to taste

2 cans (5 ounces each) tuna in water (thoroughly drained)

1 leftover hardboiled egg from Day 11 Lunch (chopped)

1/4 cup (1 ounce) shredded cheddar cheese

- For the dressing, in a medium bowl, mash cottage cheese with a fork until smooth. Add sour cream, heavy cream, bell pepper and chives, season to taste with salt and pepper and mix until thoroughly combined.

- Crumble tuna with a fork. Stir tuna and eggs into dressing, adding more heavy cream as needed to reach desired consistency.

- Sprinkle cheddar cheese over tuna salad and serve immediately. Enjoy!

PER SERVING: Calories: 179; Fat: 10g; Protein: 22g; Carbs: 3g; Fiber: 0g
Net Carbs: 3g; Fat 50% / Protein 46% / Carbs 4%

Day 13 Dinner: Turkey Zucchini Boats

Serves: 6 (plus 2 leftover portions) / Preparation time: 20 minutes / Cooking time: 40 minutes

For a Mexican flavor, use colby and jack cheeses instead of the mozzarella and Parmesan, and use chili powder and cumin in place of the Italian herb blend.

3 pounds ground turkey	3 eggs (beaten)
1 tablespoon onion powder	1 tablespoon Italian herb blend
1 tablespoon garlic powder	1 cup (4 ounces) shredded mozzarella cheese (divided)
1 teaspoon salt, plus more to taste	3 medium zucchini
1/2 teaspoon freshly ground black pepper, plus more to taste	1/4 cup (1 ounce) grated Parmesan cheese

- Preheat oven to 350°F. Spray a glass 13" x 9" baking pan with nonstick cooking spray and set aside.

- Crumble ground turkey in a large nonstick skillet over medium-high heat. Add onion powder, garlic powder, salt and pepper and cook until meat is no longer pink, about 10 minutes, stirring frequently. Drain and discard fat. Remove about 2/3 of the ground turkey from the skillet and set aside.

- For the filling, thoroughly mix eggs, Italian herb blend and half of the mozzarella cheese into the into the ground turkey in the skillet.

- Cut stems and ends off of zucchini. Cut zucchini in half lengthwise, scrape out seeds and discard. Scrape out enough flesh from zucchini halves to leave shells about 1/2" thick. Place zucchini shells in prepared pan.

- Dice removed zucchini flesh, stir into the filling and season to taste with salt and pepper. Spoon filling into zucchini shells and sprinkle with Parmesan cheese and remaining mozzarella cheese. Bake zucchini boats until cheese is melted and zucchini is tender, 25-30 minutes. Serve zucchini boats immediately. Divide reserved ground turkey into 2 portions, let cool, cover and refrigerate for later use. Enjoy!

PER SERVING: Calories: 290; Fat: 19g; Protein: 25g; Carbs: 5g; Fiber: 1g Net Carbs: 4g; Fat 59% / Protein 34% / Carbs 7%

Day 14 Breakfast: Sausage, Egg & Cheese Slices

Serves: 4 / Preparation time: 10 minutes / Cooking time: 10 minutes

Scrambled eggs, melted cheese and leftover slices of sausage-style pork meat loaf layer together to form the savory, gooey slices of this breakfast dish.

1 tablespoon vegetable oil

6 eggs (lightly beaten)

1/4 cup heavy cream

1 leftover meat loaf from Day 13 Breakfast (sliced)

1/2 cup (4 ounces) shredded cheddar cheese

- Heat oil in a large nonstick skillet over medium-high heat.

- Beat eggs and heavy cream and season to taste with salt and pepper. Arrange meat loaf slices in a single layer in skillet. Reduce heat, cover skillet and cook until eggs are nearly set, 5 to 6 minutes.

- Using a plastic spatula, cut eggs between meat loaf slices and flip all portions over. Sprinkle cheese over meat loaf slices, cover skillet and cook until cheese is melted, 2 to 3 minutes. Serve immediately and enjoy!

PER SERVING: Calories: 411; Fat: 32g; Protein: 28g; Carbs: 1g; Fiber: 0g
Net Carbs: 1g; Fat 70% / Protein 27% / Carbs 3%

Day 14 Lunch: Nutty Swiss Bites

Serves: 4 / Preparation time: 40 minutes

For extra flavor reminiscent of classic fondue, add a tablespoon of dry white wine to the cheese mixture.

1 package (3 ounces) cream cheese (softened)

1 tablespoon butter (softened)

1 leftover portion bacon drippings from Day 10 Breakfast

1 cup (4 ounces) shredded Swiss cheese

1 leftover portion bacon from Day 10 Breakfast (finely chopped)

1 teaspoon garlic powder

1/4 cup chopped walnuts (toasted)

- In a medium bowl, beat cream cheese, butter and bacon drippings with an electric hand mixer until smooth. Add Swiss cheese, bacon and garlic powder and beat until thoroughly combined.

- Refrigerate cheese mixture until firm, about 30 minutes.

- Form cheese mixture into 12 balls and roll in chopped walnuts to coat. Serve immediately and enjoy!

PER SERVING: Calories: 285; Fat: 26g; Protein: 11g; Carbs: 2g; Fiber: 1g Net Carbs: 1g; Fat 82% / Protein 15% / Carbs 3%

Day 14 Dinner: Avocado Egg Salad Wraps

Serves: 2 / Preparation time: 10 minutes

For a creamier egg salad, choose a ripe avocado and mash it slightly as you stir. If you'd prefer not to serve this dish as wraps, just tear up the lettuce, arrange on two plates and top with scoops of the egg salad.

4 leftover hard boiled eggs from Day 12 Lunch (coarsely chopped)

1 avocado (pitted, peeled, diced)

1 lime (zested, juiced)

2 tablespoons chopped fresh cilantro leaves

1/4 teaspoon chili powder

1/4 teaspoon salt, plus more to taste

1/4 teaspoon freshly ground black pepper, plus more to taste

4 large green lettuce leaves

- Mix eggs, avocado, lime juice, lime zest, cilantro, chili powder, salt and pepper until thoroughly combined.

- Layer pairs of lettuce leaves together and top each pair of leaves with half of the egg salad. Roll up lettuce leaves around egg salad, secure with decorative toothpicks if desired and serve immediately. Enjoy!

PER SERVING: Calories: 308; Fat: 24g; Protein: 15g; Carbs: 9g; Fiber: 6g Net Carbs: 3g; Fat 70% / Protein 19% / Carbs 11%

Day 15 Breakfast: Turkey Skillet

Serves: 4 / Preparation time: 5 minutes / Cooking time: 15 minutes

Garnish each serving of this savory breakfast dish with a sprinkling of grated cheese, or a dollop of sour cream or guacamole.

1 portion leftover ground turkey from Day 13 Dinner

1 can (8 ounces) tomato sauce

4 eggs

Salt and freshly ground black pepper, to taste

- Mix turkey and tomato sauce in a medium nonstick skillet over medium heat, season to taste with salt and pepper and cook until thoroughly combined and heated through.

- Make 4 wells in the turkey mixture. Crack 1 egg into each well and season eggs to taste with salt and pepper.

- Cover skillet and cook until egg whites are opaque and yolks are cooked to desired doneness, 5 to 10 minutes. Serve immediately and enjoy!

PER SERVING: Calories: 234; Fat: 12g; Protein: 28g; Carbs: 5g; Fiber: 1g Net Carbs: 4g; Fat 46% / Protein 48% / Carbs 6%

Day 15 Lunch: Curry Deviled Eggs

Serves: 4 / Preparation time: 20 minutes

For a decorative presentation, use a pastry bag fitted with a star tip to pipe the yolk mixture into the egg white halves.

8 leftover hard boiled eggs from Day 11 Lunch

1 package (3 ounces) cream cheese (softened)

3 tablespoons sour cream

1 teaspoon white vinegar

1 teaspoon mild curry powder

1/2 teaspoon ground mustard

Salt and freshly ground black pepper, to taste

Fresh cilantro, for garnish

- Cut eggs in half lengthwise with a sharp knife and remove yolks. Arrange egg white halves on a serving plate and set aside.

- In a medium bowl, mash egg yolks, cream cheese and sour cream with a fork until combined. Add vinegar, curry powder and ground mustard, season to taste with salt and pepper and continue mashing until smooth and thoroughly combined.

- Scoop yolk mixture into egg whites with a spoon and garnish with cilantro leaves to serve. Enjoy!

PER SERVING: Calories: 248; Fat: 20g; Protein: 15g; Carbs: 2g; Fiber: 0g Net Carbs: 2g; Fat 73% / Protein 24% / Carbs 3%

Day 15 Dinner: Hoisin Burgers

Serves: 4 / Preparation time: 10 minutes / Cooking time: 10 minutes

Hoisin sauce is a common Chinese condiment used with roasted or grilled meat. If you prefer a more traditional American barbecue flavor, use sliced onions instead of the bell pepper and 1/4 cup barbecue sauce instead of the hoisin sauce, soy sauce and ground ginger.

- 1 tablespoon vegetable oil
- 1 red bell pepper (sliced)
- 3 tablespoons hoisin sauce
- 1 tablespoon soy sauce
- 1 teaspoon ground ginger
- 4 leftover burgers from Day 10 Dinner

- Heat oil in a large nonstick skillet and sauté bell pepper until softened, stirring occasionally, about 5 minutes.

- Add hoisin sauce, soy sauce and ginger to skillet and stir until thoroughly combined.

- Place burgers in skillet and turn to coat. Cover skillet, reduce heat to low and cook until burgers are heated through, about 5 minutes. Arrange burgers on plates, top with the sauce and serve immediately. Enjoy!

PER SERVING: Calories: 287; Fat: 19g; Protein: 22g; Carbs: 8g; Fiber: 1g Net Carbs: 7g; Fat 60% / Protein 31% / Carbs 9%

Day 16 Breakfast: Spinach Frittata with Bacon

Serves: 4 / Preparation time: 15 minutes / Cooking time: 35 minutes

Increase the calorie count in this recipe to about 340 and the fat count to 27 grams by substituting heavy cream for the sour cream. This boosts the fat percentage to about 71%.

1 teaspoon butter

1 leftover portion bacon drippings from Day 10 Breakfast

1 bag (10 ounces) fresh baby spinach leaves

8 eggs (lightly beaten)

1/2 cup sour cream

1 leftover portion bacon from Day 10 Breakfast

Freshly ground black pepper, to taste

1/2 cup (2 ounces) grated Provolone cheese

- Preheat oven to 375°F. Grease a casserole dish with butter and set aside.

- Melt bacon drippings in a large nonstick skillet over medium heat and cook spinach until wilted. Remove skillet from heat and set aside.

- In a large bowl, whisk eggs, sour cream and bacon. Add spinach, season to taste with pepper, stir until combined and pour into prepared casserole dish.

- Sprinkle cheese over egg mixture and bake until eggs are set and cheese is melted and lightly browned, about 30 minutes. Serve frittata immediately and enjoy!

PER SERVING: Calories: 303; Fat: 22g; Protein: 21g; Carbs: 5g; Fiber: 2g Net Carbs: 3g; Fat 65% / Protein 27% / Carbs 8%

Day 16 Lunch: Asparagus Mimosa

Serves: 3 / Preparation time: 10 minutes / Cooking time: 10 minutes

Using frozen asparagus in this recipe is not recommended. If asparagus isn't in season, try substituting fresh broccoli or leeks, cut into long spears, for the asparagus.

1 pound fresh asparagus spears (about 12 medium spears)

1 teaspoon salt, plus more to taste

3 tablespoons lemon juice

1 teaspoon Dijon mustard

1/4 cup extra virgin olive oil

Freshly ground black pepper, to taste

4 leftover hard boiled eggs from Day 12 Lunch (halved)

2 tablespoons (about 1/2 ounce) freshly grated Parmesan cheese

- Trim and peel asparagus spears as necessary and place in a large skillet. Add cold water to skillet to cover asparagus, add salt and heat to a boil. Reduce heat and simmer until asparagus is tender, about 4 minutes. Transfer asparagus to an ice-water bath, drain and pat dry.

- Meanwhile, for the dressing, whisk lemon juice and Dijon mustard. Add olive oil in a thin stream, whisking constantly, until emulsified. Season dressing to taste with salt and pepper.

- Arrange asparagus spears on 3 plates, season to taste with salt and pepper and drizzle with dressing. Press egg halves through a metal mesh strainer over asparagus, sprinkle with Parmesan cheese and serve immediately. Enjoy!

PER SERVING: Calories: 294; Fat: 27g; Protein: 11g; Carbs: 3g; Fiber: 1g Net Carbs: 2g; Fat 83% / Protein 15% / Carbs 2%

Day 16 Dinner: Country-Style Ribs

Serves: 4 (plus 2 leftover portions) / Preparation time: 30 minutes (plus refrigeration time if desired) / Cooking time: 20 minutes

Using a little bit of sugar in a rib rub helps form the savory browned crust on the outer surface of the grilled meat. And since some of the sugar melts and drips off the meat during grilling, you'd be consuming less than 10 grams of carbs by eating the entire batch!

1 tablespoon brown sugar

1 tablespoon garlic power

1 tablespoon onion powder

1 tablespoon paprika

2 teaspoons chili powder

1 teaspoon salt

1 teaspoon freshly ground black pepper

1/2 teaspoon cayenne pepper, plus more to taste

6 pounds boneless pork ribs

Low carb barbecue sauce, as desired

- Mix brown sugar, garlic powder, onion powder, paprika, chili powder, salt, pepper and cayenne pepper and rub all over ribs. If desired, cover ribs and refrigerate for 30 minutes to 4 hours.

- Brush grill grate with canola oil. Preheat grill to medium-high heat.

- Place ribs on grill and grill for 8 to 10 minutes. Turn ribs over and grill until internal temperature of ribs reaches 145°F, about 8 to 10 minutes more.

- Serve about 1/3 of the ribs with sauce of choice as desired. Let remaining ribs cool, cover and refrigerate for later use. Enjoy!

PER SERVING: Calories: 242; Fat: 15g; Protein: 25g; Carbs: 1g; Fiber: 0g Net Carbs: 1g; Fat 56% / Protein 41% / Carbs 3%

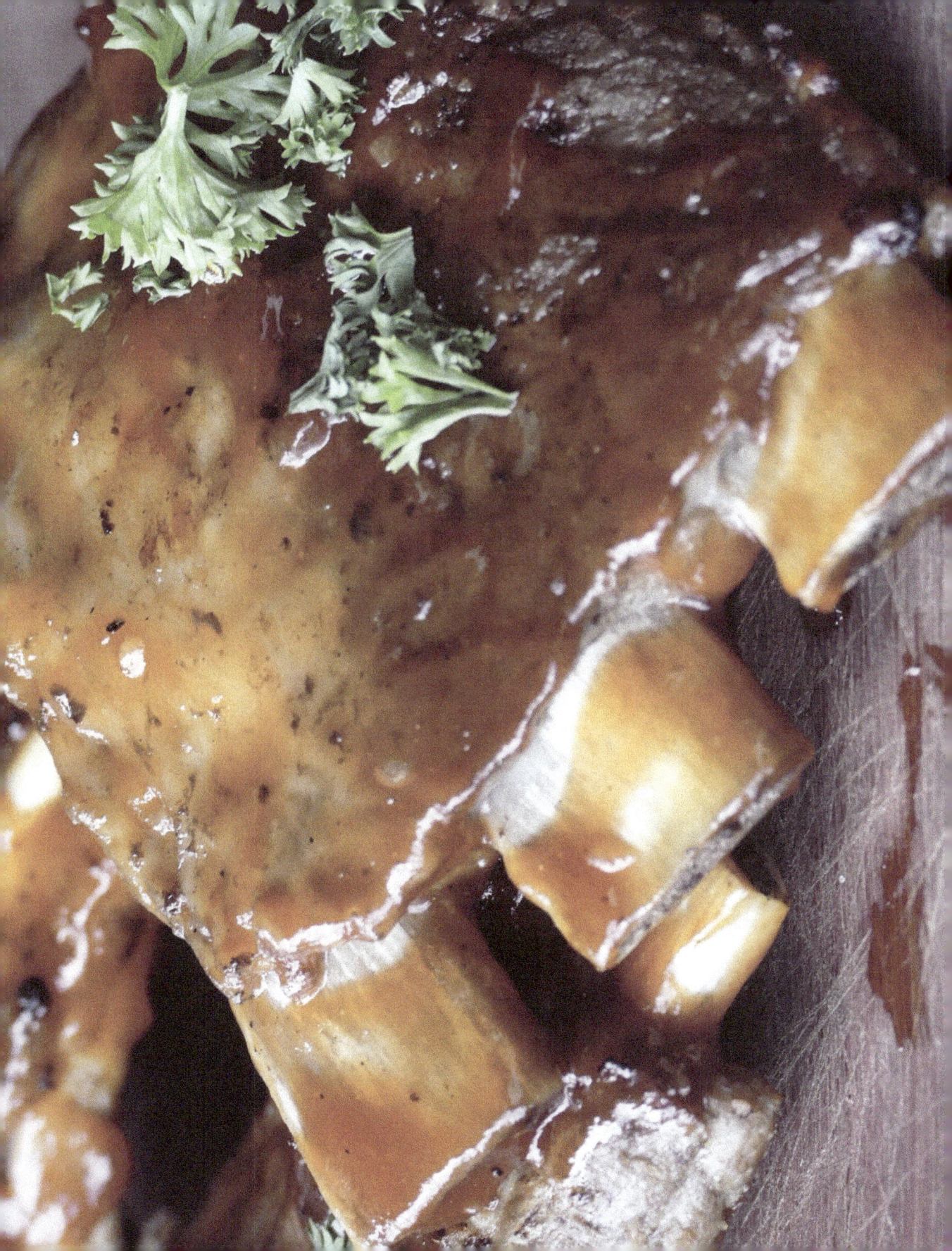

Day 17 Breakfast: Bacon-Wrapped Sausage

Serves: 8 / Preparation time: 15 minutes / Cooking time: 20 minutes

What could possibly go better with breakfast meat than more breakfast meat?

1 tablespoon dried dill

1 leftover meat loaf from Day 13 Breakfast (sliced)

1 package (16 ounces) bacon

- Sprinkle dill all over meat loaf slices.

- Wrap each slice of meat loaf in 2 slices of bacon.

- Fry 3 to 4 bacon-wrapped slices in a large nonstick skillet over medium-high heat until bacon is done to desired crispness, turning as necessary, 4 to 8 minutes per side. Drain cooked slices on paper towels.

- Repeat with remaining slices. Serve immediately and enjoy!

PER SERVING: Calories: 175; Fat: 13g; Protein: 13g; Carbs: 0g; Fiber: 0g Net Carbs: 0g; Fat 68% / Protein 32% / Carbs 0%

Day 17 Lunch: Grilled Cheese Sandwiches

Serves: 2 (plus 2 leftover portions) / Preparation time: 30 minutes / Cooking time: 45 minutes

These sandwiches are so gooey and tasty, you won't even miss the bread.

1 large head cauliflower (cut into florets)

1 tablespoon water

3 eggs

3/4 cup (3 ounces) grated Parmesan cheese

1/2 teaspoon salt

1 tablespoon butter

2 slices (1 ounce each) colby jack cheese

- For the cauliflower slices, pulse cauliflower in a food processor until grainy. Transfer cauliflower to a bowl and sprinkle with water. Cover bowl and cook cauliflower in the microwave for 2 minutes. Stir cauliflower and cook 2 minutes more. Let cauliflower cool.

- Preheat oven to 350°F.

- Mix eggs, Parmesan and salt into cooled cauliflower until thoroughly combined.

- Line a baking sheet with parchment paper. Scoop cauliflower onto baking sheet in 12 portions and form each into a square about 1/2" thick. Bake slices for about 15 minutes. Carefully turn slices over and bake 15 minutes more.

- Melt butter in a large nonstick skillet over medium heat. Place 2 slices in skillet and top each with cheese and another slice. Cover skillet and cook until sandwiches are golden and cheese is melted, turning over as necessary, about 10 minutes total. Serve sandwiches immediately. Let remaining 8 slices cool, layer in parchment paper, place in a covered container and freeze for later use. Enjoy!

PER SERVING: Calories: 278; Fat: 22g; Protein: 17g; Carbs: 4g; Fiber: 2g Net Carbs: 2g; Fat 71% / Protein 24% / Carbs 5%

Day 17 Dinner: Creamy White Chili

Serves: 4 / Preparation time: 15 minutes / Cooking time: 20 minutes

Avocado slices, jalapeno peppers or halved cherry tomatoes would make attractive (and tasty!) garnish for bowls of this unique chili.

1 tablespoon butter

1 small onion (minced)

1 small head cauliflower (riced)

2 garlic cloves (minced)

1 leftover portion ground turkey from Day 13 Dinner

2 cups chicken stock

1/2 cup sour cream

1 package (3 ounces) cream cheese

1 can (4 1/2 ounces) chopped green chilies (drained)

2 teaspoons cumin

1 teaspoon ground mustard

1 teaspoon dried thyme

1/2 teaspoon celery salt

1/2 teaspoon salt, plus more to taste

1/4 teaspoon freshly ground black pepper, plus more to taste

- Melt butter in a large saucepan over medium heat and sauté onion and cauliflower until softened, stirring occasionally, about 5 minutes. Add garlic and sauté about 1 minute more, stirring constantly. Add turkey and stir until combined.

- Add chicken stock, sour cream, cream cheese, green chilies, cumin, mustard, thyme, celery salt, salt and pepper to saucepan and stir until combined. Heat chili to a simmer, stirring constantly.

- Reduce heat to low, cover pan and simmer chili for about 10 minutes, stirring occasionally. Season chili to taste with salt and pepper and serve immediately. Enjoy!

**PER SERVING: Calories: 349; Fat: 24g; Protein: 26g; Carbs: 8g; Fiber: 2g
Net Carbs: 6g; Fat 62% / Protein 30% / Carbs 8%**

Day 18 Breakfast: Keto Coconut Pancakes

Serves: 4 (plus 2 leftover portions) / Preparation time: 15 minutes / Cooking time: 20 minutes

Using maple extract mimics the flavor of pancake syrup without adding carbs. If you prefer, you could use vanilla extract or coconut extract instead.

1/4 cup heavy cream

12 eggs

3/4 cup sour cream

1/2 cup butter (melted)

1 teaspoon maple extract

3/4 cup coconut flour

1 1/2 teaspoons baking powder

Powdered sweetener of choice equivalent to 3 tablespoons sugar

1/4 teaspoon salt

Coconut oil (for frying)

1/4 cup unsweetened flaked coconut (toasted)

- In a small bowl, whip cream with an electric hand mixer until stiff peaks form. Cover bowl and refrigerate until serving.

- In a large bowl, beat eggs, sour cream, butter and maple extract until thoroughly combined. In a small bowl, mix coconut flour, baking powder, sweetener and salt until thoroughly combined. Add dry ingredients to wet ingredients and mix just until combined. Add water 1 tablespoon at a time as needed to reach desired consistency.

- Melt 1 tablespoon coconut oil on a large nonstick griddle over medium heat. Pour batter onto griddle in 1/4 cup portions and cook until surface is bubbly, about 3 minutes. Turn pancakes and cook until lightly browned on the bottom, about 2 minutes. Remove finished pancakes to a serving plate and repeat with remaining batter.

- Divide pancakes in to 3 portions. Top 1 portion of pancakes with whipped cream, sprinkle with coconut and serve immediately. Let remaining 2 portions of pancakes cool, cover and refrigerate for later use. Enjoy!

PER SERVING: Calories: 289; Fat: 25g; Protein: 9g; Carbs: 8g; Fiber: 4g Net Carbs: 4g; Fat 78% / Protein 12% / Carbs 10%

Day 18 Lunch: Lemon Butter Tilapia

Serves: 4 (plus 2 leftover portions) / Preparation time: 10 minutes / Cooking time: 20 minutes

For a subtle change of taste, use lime juice instead of lemon juice.

1/4 cup butter

8 garlic cloves (minced)

1/4 cup lemon juice

1 teaspoon Old Bay Seasoning

Salt and freshly ground black pepper, to taste

1/4 cup fresh chopped parsley leaves

12 tilapia fillets (about 6 ounces each)

- Preheat oven to 400°F. Spray a large rimmed baking pan with nonstick cooking spray and set aside.

- Melt butter in a small saucepan over low heat. Add garlic and sauté for about 2 minutes, stirring occasionally. Remove pan from heat, add lemon juice and stir until combined.

- Arrange tilapia fillets in a single layer on prepared baking sheet, sprinkle with Old Bay Seasoning and season to taste with salt and pepper. Pour butter mixture over tilapia fillets and sprinkle with parsley leaves.

- Bake until fillets are cooked through and flaky, about 15 minutes. Serve 4 fillets immediately as desired. Let remaining fillets cool, cover and refrigerate for later use. Enjoy!

PER SERVING: Calories: 148; Fat: 6g; Protein: 23g; Carbs: 1g; Fiber: 0g Net Carbs: 1g; Fat 36% / Protein 62% / Carbs 2%

Day 18 Dinner: Pulled Pork

Serves: 4 / Preparation time: 15 minutes / Cooking time: 60 minutes

Serve this savory pulled pork alongside some vinegar-and-oil cole slaw for a delicious contrast in flavor and texture.

- 1 tablespoon vegetable oil
- 1 medium onion (sliced)
- 1/4 cup water
- 1 tablespoon Worcestershire sauce
- 1 tablespoon chili powder
- 1 tablespoon apple cider vinegar
- 1 leftover portion country-style ribs from Day 16 Dinner
- Low carb barbecue sauce, as desired

- Heat oil in a large nonstick skillet over medium heat and sauté onion until caramelized, stirring occasionally, 7 to 8 minutes. Add water, Worcestershire sauce, chili powder and vinegar and stir until combined.

- Arrange ribs in a single layer over mixture in skillet. Reduce heat, cover skillet and cook until ribs are tender and falling apart, 45 minutes to 1 hour.

- Shred ribs with a fork and serve with barbecue sauce as desired. Enjoy!

PER SERVING: Calories: 256; Fat: 15g; Protein: 25g; Carbs: 4g; Fiber: 1g Net Carbs: 3g; Fat 53% / Protein 39% / Carbs 8%

Day 19 Breakfast: Keto Vanilla Yogurt

Serves: 2 (plus 3 leftover portions) / Preparation time: 10 minutes

Sweetened packaged yogurt is generally pretty high in carbs. This keto version should satisfy your cravings! For a fluffier version, whip the cream first.

2 cups sour cream

1/4 cup heavy cream

1 teaspoon vanilla extract

Sweetener of choice equal to 1/4 cup sugar

- In a medium bowl, beat sour cream, heavy cream and vanilla extract with an electric hand mixer until combined.

- While mixing, add sweetener in a slow and steady stream. Continue mixing until sweetener is dissolved.

- Divide yogurt into 4 portions and serve 1 portion immediately. Cover remaining 3 portions and refrigerate for later use. Enjoy!

PER SERVING: Calories: 199; Fat: 20g; Protein: 3g; Carbs: 4g; Fiber: 0g Net Carbs: 0g; Fat 90% / Protein 10% / Carbs 0%

Day 19 Lunch: Bacon Cheddar Sandwiches

Serves: 2 / Preparation time: 5 minutes / Cooking time: 20 minutes

You don't need to thaw the frozen slices before assembling and frying these sandwiches.

4 bacon slices

4 cauliflower slices from Day 17 Lunch

2 slices (1 ounce each) mild cheddar cheese

1 Roma tomato (sliced)

- Fry bacon in a large nonstick skillet over medium-high heat to desired doneness, 4 to 8 minutes. Remove bacon from skillet and drain on paper towels.

- Swirl skillet to evenly distribute bacon fat. Place 2 cauliflower slices in skillet and top with bacon, cheese, tomato and remaining cauliflower slices. Cover skillet and cook until sandwiches are golden and cheese is melted, turning over as necessary, about 10 minutes total. Serve sandwiches immediately and enjoy!

PER SERVING: Calories: 329; Fat: 24g; Protein: 24g; Carbs: 6g; Fiber: 2g
Net Carbs: 4g; Fat 66% / Protein 29% / Carbs 5%

Day 19 Dinner: Meatball Parmigiana

Serves: 4 (plus 2 leftover portions) / Preparation time: 20 minutes / Cooking time: 40 minutes

For extra Italian flavor, sprinkle dried basil, oregano, marjoram, thyme and/or rosemary over the meatballs in the casserole dish before topping with the marinara and mozzarella.

- 2 pounds ground beef
- 1 pound ground pork
- 1/4 cup fresh chopped parsley
- 1 1/2 cups (6 ounces) grated Parmesan cheese
- 1 cup almond flour
- 4 eggs
- 1 tablespoon dried minced onion
- 1 teaspoon salt, plus more to taste
- 1/2 teaspoon freshly ground black pepper, plus more to taste
- 1/2 teaspoon garlic powder
- 1 cup sugar-free marinara sauce
- 1 cup (4 ounces) grated mozzarella cheese

- Preheat oven to 350°F. Spray a large rimmed baking sheet with nonstick cooking spray and set aside.

- In a large bowl, knead ground beef, ground pork, parsley, Parmesan cheese, almond flour, eggs, minced onion, salt, pepper and garlic powder until thoroughly combined (do not overmix). Form meat mixture into about 60 meatballs.

- Arrange meatballs in a single layer on prepared baking sheet and bake until cooked through and lightly browned, about 20 minutes.

- Transfer about 20 meatballs to an oven-safe casserole dish. Pour marinara sauce over meatballs and sprinkle with mozzarella cheese. Bake until cheese is melted and golden, about 20 minutes. Serve meatball parmigiana immediately. Let remaining meatballs cool, divide into 2 portions, cover and refrigerate for later use. Enjoy!

PER SERVING: Calories: 242; Fat: 16g; Protein: 22g; Carbs: 1g; Fiber: 0g Net Carbs: 1g; Fat 60% / Protein 36% / Carbs 4%

Day 20 Breakfast: Pancakes with Peanut Butter Fluff

Serves: 4 / Preparation time: 15 minutes

If you can spare the carbs, a tablespoon of semisweet chocolate chips and drizzle over the topped pancakes. You'll be adding just 2 grams of carbs for a flavor reminiscent of peanut butter cups!

1/4 cup natural peanut butter

1/4 cup heavy cream

1 package (3 ounces) cream cheese (softened)

1 leftover portion pancakes from Day 18 breakfast

- In a small bowl, beat peanut butter, heavy cream and cream cheese until thoroughly combined and fluffy.
- Reheat pancakes in the microwave, top with dollops of peanut butter fluff and serve immediately. Enjoy!

PER SERVING: Calories: 430; Fat: 37g; Protein: 14g; Carbs: 10g; Fiber: 4g Net Carbs: 6g; Fat 77% / Protein 13% / Carbs 10%

Day 20 Lunch: Tilapia Cakes

Serves: 4 / Preparation time: 10 minutes / Cooking time: 20 minutes

The ginger, coriander and turmeric give these tilapia cakes an Indian flavor. Serve them with a spicy and sour cilantro and lime chutney or a creamy cucumber and mint raita.

1 leftover portion tilapia from Day 18 Lunch

4 ounces fried pork rinds (crushed to about 1/2 cup)

2 eggs (lightly beaten)

3 tablespoons minced onion

1 knob ginger (about 1", minced)

1 teaspoon chili powder

1 teaspoon ground coriander

1 teaspoon cumin

1/2 teaspoon turmeric

1/2 teaspoon salt, plus more to taste

1/2 teaspoon freshly ground black pepper, plus more to taste

Chopped fresh cilantro, for garnish

- Flake tilapia with a fork and mix with pork rinds, eggs, onion, ginger, chili powder, coriander, cumin, turmeric, salt and pepper. Divide mixture into 8 portions and form each portion into a flat round cake.

- Melt butter in a large nonstick skillet over medium-low heat and fry tilapia cakes until golden brown on both sides, about 8 minutes total, turning as necessary. Fry cakes in batches if necessary, keeping finished cakes warm. Sprinkle cakes with cilantro and serve immediately. Enjoy!

PER SERVING: Calories: 339; Fat: 17g; Protein: 43g; Carbs: 2g; Fiber: 0g Net Carbs: 2g; Fat 45% / Protein 51% / Carbs 4%

Day 20 Dinner: Shredded Pork Taco Salads

Serves: 4 / Preparation time: 30 minutes / Cooking time: 45 to 60 minutes

For extra color and flavor, sprinkle some grated Colby-jack cheese over these tasty salads.

1 tablespoon vegetable oil

1 onion (sliced)

1 green bell pepper (sliced)

1/4 cup water

1 tablespoon chili powder

1 tablespoon cumin

1 leftover portion country-style ribs from Day 16 Dinner

4 cups torn green leaf lettuce

1 tomato (diced)

1 avocado (pitted, peeled, sliced)

- Heat oil in a large nonstick skillet over medium heat and sauté onion and bell pepper until softened, stirring occasionally, 5 to 6 minutes. Add water, chili powder and cumin and stir until combined.

- Arrange ribs in a single layer over mixture in skillet. Reduce heat, cover skillet and cook until ribs are tender and falling apart, 45 minutes to 1 hour.

- Shred ribs with a fork and mix with pepper and onion. Divide lettuce among 4 salad bowls and top with tomato, shredded pork and avocado slices. Serve immediately and enjoy!

PER SERVING: Calories: 378; Fat: 26g; Protein: 27g; Carbs: 12g; Fiber: 5g Net Carbs: 7g; Fat 62% / Protein 29% / Carbs 9%

Day 21 Breakfast: Chocolate Almond Smoothies

Serves: 2 / Preparation time: 10 minutes

For extra protein and flavor, add scoops of your choice of low-carb protein powder to these smoothies.

1 leftover portion keto yogurt from Day 19 Breakfast

6 to 8 ice cubes

1 tablespoon almond butter

1/2 teaspoon almond extract

- Place all ingredients in a blender container and purée to desired consistency. Pour into 2 large glasses and serve immediately. Enjoy!

PER SERVING: Calories: 248; Fat: 25g; Protein: 4g; Carbs: 6g; Fiber: 1g Net Carbs: 5g; Fat 91% / Protein 4% / Carbs 5%

Day 21 Lunch: Ham and Swiss Panini

Serves: 2 / Preparation time: 10 minutes / Cooking time: 5 minutes

If you don't have a panini press, you can fry these sandwiches in a nonstick skillet.

1 teaspoon olive oil

4 cauliflower slices from Day 17 Lunch

2 teaspoons Dijon mustard

2 teaspoons mayonnaise

6 thin slices (about 4 ounces) smoked deli ham

2 slices (1 ounce each) Swiss cheese

Dill pickle spears, for garnish

- Brush panini press with olive oil and preheat according to manufacturer's directions.

- Spread mustard on 2 cauliflower slices. Spread mayonnaise on the other 2 cauliflower slices. Place 2 cauliflower slices in panini press with plain sides facing down. Top with ham, Swiss cheese and remaining cauliflower slices with plain sides facing up.

- Close press and cook until cheese is melted and sandwiches are crisp and golden, 3 to 5 minutes. Serve immediately with the pickle spears and enjoy!

PER SERVING: Calories: 346; Fat: 22g; Protein: 29g; Carbs: 5g; Fiber: 2g Net Carbs: 3g; Fat 57% / Protein 33% / Carbs 10%

Day 21 Dinner: Meatball Stroganoff

Serves: 4 / Preparation time: 10 minutes / Cooking time: 20 minutes

Serve these savory meatballs in their creamy sauce over mashed cauliflower or zoodles.

- 1 tablespoon vegetable oil
- 8 ounces baby bella mushrooms (sliced)
- 1 cup beef stock or broth
- 1/4 teaspoon garlic powder
- 1/4 teaspoon freshly ground black pepper, plus more to taste
- Salt, to taste
- 1 leftover portion meatballs from Day 19 Dinner
- 1/2 cup sour cream

- Heat oil in a medium nonstick skillet over medium heat and sauté mushrooms until softened, stirring frequently, about 5 minutes. Add stock, garlic powder and pepper to skillet, season to taste with salt and stir to deglaze.

- Add meatballs to skillet and cook until heated through, about 5 minutes, stirring occasionally.

- Remove skillet from heat, stir in sour cream and serve immediately. Enjoy!

PER SERVING: Calories: 335; Fat: 27g; Protein: 17g; Carbs: 8g; Fiber: 2g Net Carbs: 6g; Fat 73% / Protein 20% / Carbs 70%

Day 22 Breakfast: Berries and Cream Pancakes

Serves: 4 / Preparation time: 10 minutes

For a heartier cream topping, add a small package of cream cheese to the mixture.

1/2 cup sliced strawberries

1/2 cup raspberries

1/2 cup blueberries

1/4 cup heavy cream

1 leftover portion pancakes from Day 18 breakfast

- Mix berries in a small bowl and lightly mash with a fork. Set berries aside.
- Whip heavy cream in a small bowl with an electric hand mixer until stiff peaks form. Gently fold berries into whipped cream.
- Reheat pancakes in the microwave, top with dollops of berries and cream and serve immediately. Enjoy!

PER SERVING: Calories: 278; Fat: 22g; Protein: 9g; Carbs: 13g; Fiber: 5g Net Carbs: 8g; Fat 71% / Protein 18% / Carbs 11%

Day 22 Lunch: Kale Pesto Tilapia

Serves: 4 / Preparation time: 15 minutes

Add an extra layer of flavor to this already tasty pesto by lightly toasting the walnuts before proceeding with the recipe.

1 1/2 cups (3 ounces) fresh kale (chopped)

1/3 cup (2 ounces) chopped walnuts

1 garlic clove (minced)

1 teaspoon lemon juice

1/4 teaspoon salt, plus more to taste

1/4 teaspoon freshly ground black pepper, plus more to taste

1/4 cup extra virgin olive oil

1/4 cup (1 ounce) grated Parmesan cheese

1 leftover portion tilapia from Day 18 Lunch

- Purée kale, walnuts, garlic, lemon juice, salt and pepper in a food processor until smooth. While processing, add oil in a slow, thin stream and continue processing until smooth. Add Parmesan cheese and process just until combined.

- Reheat tilapia fillets in the microwave and serve immediately with the pesto. Enjoy!

PER SERVING: Calories: 406; Fat: 31g; Protein: 29g; Carbs: 6g; Fiber: 2g Net Carbs: 4g; Fat 69% / Protein 29% / Carbs 2%

Day 22 Dinner: Smoky Slow Cooker Chicken

Serves: 4 (plus 2 leftover portions) / Preparation time: 30 minutes / Cooking time: 5 hours

Serve this smoky chicken with roasted vegetables or buttered mashed cauliflower.

1 whole roasting chicken (about 5 pounds)

1 tablespoon butter (melted)

1 tablespoon smoked paprika

2 teaspoons salt, plus more to taste

1 teaspoon pepper, plus more to taste

1 teaspoon garlic powder

1/2 teaspoon liquid smoke

1 onion (sliced)

- Remove neck and giblets from chicken body cavity as necessary and discard. Rinse chicken inside and out with cold water and pat dry with paper towels. Brush chicken with butter. Mix smoked paprika, salt, pepper and garlic powder and rub all over chicken.

- Brush inner crock of slow cooker with liquid smoke. Scatter onion slices on bottom of crock. Set chicken in crock, cover and cook on low setting for about 5 hours.

- Carve breasts from chicken, cut into slices and serve immediately. Set remaining chicken aside and let cool. Carve thighs from chicken and shred meat with a fork. Place shredded meat and remaining chicken frame in separate containers, cover and refrigerate for later use. Enjoy!

PER SERVING: Calories: 123; Fat: 3g; Protein: 24g; Carbs: 0g; Fiber: 0g Net Carbs: 0g; Fat 22% / Protein 88% / Carbs 0%

Day 23 Breakfast: Green Smoothies

Serves: 2 / Preparation time: 10

For a stronger flavor, use fresh kale instead of the spinach. You can also add your favorite seasonings or herbs, such as basil or chili powder.

- 6 to 8 ice cubes
- 1 leftover portion keto yogurt from Day 19 Breakfast
- 1 medium cucumber (peeled, seeded, cubed)
- 1 package (10 ounces) baby spinach leaves
- 1/4 teaspoon salt
- Cayenne pepper and freshly ground black pepper, to taste

- Place all ingredients in a blender container and purée to desired consistency. Pour into 2 large glasses and serve immediately. Enjoy!

PER SERVING: Calories: 244; Fat: 21g; Protein: 8g; Carbs: 11g; Fiber: 4g Net Carbs: 7g; Fat 77% / Protein 13% / Carbs 10%

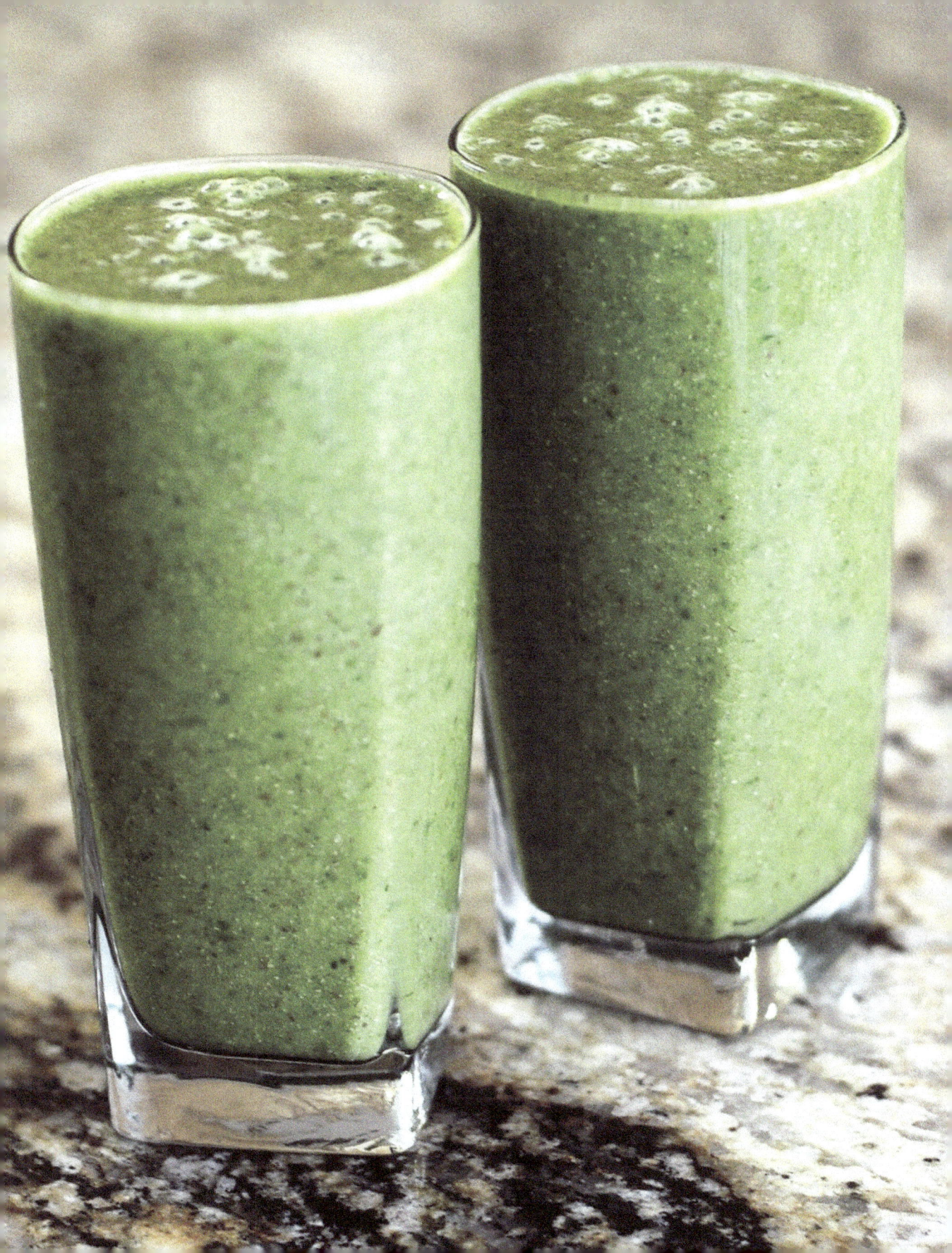

Day 23 Lunch: Buttered Zoodles

Serves: 4 (plus 2 leftover portions) / Preparation time: 45 minutes / Cooking time: 2 to 3 minutes

"Zoodle" is a mash-up of the words "zucchini" and "noodle." You could use other summer squash in this recipe instead of the zucchini, but then you'd have to call them squoodles!

2 pounds zucchini (about 8 medium)

2 teaspoons salt, plus more to taste

1 tablespoon vegetable oil

1 tablespoon butter

- Cut stems and ends from zucchini and discard. Cut zucchini into thin noodle-like strips with a spiralizer, mandoline or vegetable peeler.

- Place zucchini in a colander, sprinkle with salt and let stand for about 30 minutes to draw out moisture.

- Blot zucchini as dry as possible with paper towels.

- Heat oil in a large nonstick skillet and sauté zoodles until crisp-tender, stirring frequently, 2 to 3 minutes.

- Divide zoodles into 3 portions. Toss 1 portion zoodles with butter, season to taste with salt and serve immediately. Let remaining 2 portions of zoodles cool, cover and refrigerate for later use. Enjoy!

PER SERVING: Calories: 71; Fat: 7g; Protein: 2g; Carbs: 2g; Fiber: 1g Net Carbs: 1g; Fat 88% / Protein 11% / Carbs 1%

Day 23 Dinner: BBQ Meatballs

Serves: 4 / Preparation time: 10 minutes / Cooking time: 3 to 4 minutes

If you have a favorite low-carb barbecue sauce, feel free to use it in place of the sauce in this recipe.

2 tablespoons reduced-sugar ketchup

2 tablespoons heavy cream

2 tablespoons Italian salad dressing

1/4 teaspoon liquid smoke

1/4 teaspoon onion powder

1/4 teaspoon freshly ground black pepper

1 leftover portion meatballs from Day 19 Dinner

- Preheat oven broiler. Spray an oven-proof casserole dish with nonstick cooking spray.

- For the sauce, whisk ketchup, heavy cream, salad dressing, liquid smoke, onion powder and pepper. Toss sauce with meatballs to coat.

- Arrange meatballs in a single layer in prepared casserole dish and broil, watching carefully, until meatballs are heated through and lightly browned, 3 to 4 minutes. Serve immediately and enjoy!

PER SERVING: Calories: 293; Fat: 23g; Protein: 14g; Carbs: 7g; Fiber: 1g Net Carbs: 6g; Fat 71% / Protein 19% / Carbs 10%

Day 24 Breakfast: Bacon and Egg Cups

Serves: 4 (plus 2 leftover portions) / Preparation time: 10 minutes / Cooking time: 40 minutes

These cups are not really meant to be served as an "on-the-go" meal. They're easier to eat with a fork and knife.

1 package (12 ounces) bacon

12 eggs

Salt and freshly ground black pepper, to taste

- Preheat oven to 350°F.

- Partially cook bacon slices in a nonstick skillet over medium-high heat (bacon should remain pliable). Drain bacon and use fat to grease the wells of a 12-cup muffin pan.

- Line bottoms and sides of muffin wells with bacon slices. Crack one egg into each bacon-lined well and season to taste with salt and pepper. Pierce egg yolks with a fork and stir gently.

- Bake cups until eggs are set, 25-30 minutes. Serve 4 cups immediately. Let remaining 8 cups cool, cover and refrigerate for later use. Enjoy!

PER SERVING: Calories: 142; Fat: 11g; Protein: 9g; Carbs: 1g; Fiber: 0g Net Carbs: 1g; Fat 70% / Protein 25% / Carbs 5%

Day 24 Lunch: Keto Quesadilla

Serves: 2 (plus 2 leftover portions) / Preparation time: 10 minutes / Cooking time: 20 minutes

Note that for this recipe, it's okay if a bit of egg yolk gets mixed in with the whites since you won't be whipping the whites like you would for a meringue.

- 12 eggs
- 1 1/2 cup water
- 6 tablespoons coconut flour
- 3/4 teaspoon baking powder
- 3/4 teaspoon onion powder
- 3/4 teaspoon garlic powder
- 3/4 teaspoon salt
- 6 tablespoons vegetable oil
- 1/2 cup (2 ounces) shredded pepper jack cheese
- 1 avocado (halved, pitted, sliced)

- Separate eggs. Place yolks in a covered container and refrigerate for later use.

- For the tortillas, whisk egg whites with water until thoroughly combined. Add coconut flour, baking powder, onion powder, garlic powder and salt to egg white mixture and whisk until smooth. Batter will be thin.

- Heat 1 tablespoon vegetable oil in a large nonstick skillet over medium-high heat. Pour about 1/3 cup batter into skillet, spreading as evenly and thinly as possible. Fry tortilla until golden brown on both sides, turning as necessary, about 3 minutes total. Remove tortilla from skillet and repeat with remaining vegetable oil and batter, finishing with 8 tortillas.

- For the quesadilla, return 1 tortilla to skillet and top with cheese and another tortilla. Fry until cheese is melted, about 1 minute. Cut quesadilla into wedges and serve immediately with the avocado slices. Let remaining 6 tortillas cool, cover and refrigerate for later use. Enjoy!

PER SERVING: Calories: 348; Fat: 28g; Protein: 16g; Carbs: 12g; Fiber: 10g Net Carbs: 2g; Fat 72% / Protein 18% / Carbs 10%

Day 24 Dinner: Smoky Chicken Soup

Serves: 6 / Preparation time: 1 hour / Cooking time: 2 hours

If you don't have New Mexico chili powder (made up exclusively of ground dried Hatch chilies), you can substitute an equal amount of ancho chili powder, or about half the amount of chipotle chili powder.

- Leftover chicken frame from Day 22 Dinner
- 8 cups water
- 1 1/2 teaspoons garlic powder
- 1 1/2 teaspoons onion powder
- 2 teaspoons salt (divided)
- 1 teaspoon freshly ground black pepper (divided)
- 1 tablespoon vegetable oil
- 1 onion (diced)
- 1 jalapeño pepper (seeded, diced)
- 4 garlic cloves (minced)
- 2 tablespoons ground cumin
- 2 tablespoons New Mexico chili powder
- 2 cans (14.5 ounces each) fire-roasted diced tomatoes (undrained)
- 1/2 cup sour cream
- 1/2 cup (2 ounces) crumbled queso fresco
- 1 lime (cut into wedges)

- Place chicken frame, water, garlic powder, onion powder, 1 teaspoon salt and 1/2 teaspoon black pepper in a stock pot and heat to a boil, skimming foam as necessary. Reduce heat, cover pot and simmer for 1 1/2 hours.

- Remove chicken from broth and let stand until cool enough to handle. Shred meat from bones and set aside. Discard bones and skin. Strain broth into a large container and set aside. Discard strained solids.

- Rinse and dry stock pot. Heat oil in pot and sauté onion and jalapeño pepper until softened, about 5 minutes, stirring frequently. Add garlic and sauté about 1 minute more, stirring constantly. Add cumin, chili powder and remaining 1/2 teaspoon black pepper and cook until fragrant, about 1 minute, stirring constantly.

- Pour about 1 cup broth into pot and stir to deglaze. Add remaining broth, undrained tomatoes and remaining 1 teaspoon salt to pot and stir to combine. Heat soup to a boil, stirring occasionally. Reduce heat, cover and simmer soup for 30 minutes, stirring occasionally.

- Ladle soup into bowls to serve and pass the sour cream, queso fresco and lime wedges on the side. Enjoy!

PER SERVING: Calories: 216; Fat: 11g; Protein: 22g; Carbs: 7g; Fiber: 2g Net Carbs: 5g; Fat 46% / Protein 41% / Carbs 13%

Day 25 Breakfast: Strawberry Cheesecake Smoothies

Serves: 2 / Preparation time: 10 minutes

Substitute raspberries and/or blackberries for some or all of the strawberries in this recipe for a slight reduction in carbs, but a big change of taste!

- 1 leftover portion keto yogurt from Day 19 Breakfast
- 6 to 8 ice cubes
- 1/2 cup sliced strawberries
- 2 tablespoons cream cheese (softened)
- 3 cups unsweetened almond milk
- 1/4 teaspoon vanilla extract

- Place all ingredients in a blender container and purée to desired consistency. Pour into 2 large glasses and serve immediately. Enjoy!

PER SERVING: Calories: 260; Fat: 25g; Protein: 4g; Carbs: 7g; Fiber: 1g Net Carbs: 6g; Fat 87% / Protein 6% / Carbs 7%

Day 25 Lunch: Garlic Shrimp Zoodles Alfredo

Serves: 4 / Preparation time: 10 minutes / Cooking time: 15 minutes

If you've been on a keto diet for any length of time, it's likely that you've already tried zoodles. They don't taste anything like pasta, but they stand in for it very nicely in saucy, savory dishes like this one.

- 1 leftover portion zoodles from Day 23 Lunch
- 2 tablespoons butter (divided)
- 1 pound baby shrimp
- 4 garlic cloves (minced)
- 1 package (3 ounces) cream cheese
- 1/2 cup (2 ounces) grated Parmesan cheese
- 1/2 cup heavy cream
- 1/2 teaspoon dried red pepper flakes
- Salt and freshly ground black pepper, to taste

- Place zoodles in a colander and let drain while preparing the rest of the recipe.
- Melt 1 tablespoon butter in a large nonstick skillet over medium heat and sauté shrimp and garlic until shrimp is bright pink and garlic is softened, about 2 minutes, stirring frequently. Remove shrimp mixture from skillet and set aside.
- Cut cream cheese into chunks, add to skillet with the Parmesan cheese, heavy cream and remaining 1 tablespoon butter and stir until the cheeses are melted and smooth.
- Add shrimp, zoodles and red pepper flakes to skillet, season to taste with salt and pepper and stir until heated through. Serve immediately and enjoy!

PER SERVING: Calories: 446; Fat: 36g; Protein: 28g; Carbs: 5g; Fiber: 3g Net Carbs: 2g; Fat 73% / Protein 25% / Carbs 2%

Day 25 Dinner: Egg Yolk Frittata

Serves: 4 / Preparation time: 15 minutes / Cooking time: 10 minutes

Since you're only using egg yolks, this frittata will be fairly dense. Whisking the egg mixture incorporates air, helping your finished frittata attain a fluffier texture. If you prefer, you could use an electric hand mixer.

2 tablespoons chopped fresh chives

1/4 cup heavy cream

1 package (3 ounces) cream cheese (softened)

1/4 cup sour cream

12 leftover egg yolks from Day 24 Lunch

1 tablespoon butter

- For the spread, mix chives into cream cheese until thoroughly combined. Set spread aside.
- For the frittata, whisk egg yolks, heavy cream and sour cream until thickened and fluffy.
- Melt butter in a large nonstick skillet over medium heat. Add egg yolk mixture, cover skillet and cook until nearly set on the top, 5 to 6 minutes.
- Carefully turn frittata and cook until eggs are fully set, about 4 minutes more.
- Transfer frittata to a serving plate and cut into wedges. Serve frittata with chive cream cheese spread on the side and enjoy!

PER SERVING: Calories: 346; Fat: 32g; Protein: 11g; Carbs: 4g; Fiber: 0g
Net Carbs: 4g; Fat 83% / Protein 13% / Carbs 4%

Day 26 Breakfast: Veggie Bacon Egg Cups

Serves: 4 / Preparation time: 10 minutes / Cooking time: 10 minutes

Using a sliced green bell pepper in place of the zucchini in this recipe will not change the carb count at all, but it will definitely change the taste. Give it a try next time!

1 medium zucchini

1 tablespoon butter

1 onion (sliced)

4 leftover bacon and egg cups from Day 24 Breakfast

- Cut stem and end from zucchini and shred with a box grater or food processor.

- Melt butter in a large nonstick skillet and sauté zucchini and onion until softened and lightly browned, stirring frequently, 7 to 8 minutes.

- Reheat bacon and egg cups in the microwave, top with zucchini mixture and serve immediately. Enjoy!

PER SERVING: Calories: 178; Fat: 14g; Protein: 9g; Carbs: 4g; Fiber: 1g Net Carbs: 3g; Fat 71% / Protein 20% / Carbs 9%

Day 26 Lunch: Avocado Salad

Serves: 4 / Preparation time: 20 minutes / Cooking time: 11 minutes

If you prefer a creamier, guacamole-style salad, use soft, ripe avocados. For a chunkier salad, use firmer avocados.

2 bacon slices (diced)

1 tablespoon minced onion

1 garlic clove (minced)

2 avocados (halved, pitted, diced)

1 lime (zested, juiced)

1 Roma tomato (diced)

Salt, freshly ground black pepper and cayenne pepper, to taste

2 tablespoons sour cream

2 leftover tortillas from Day 24 Lunch

- Sauté bacon in a small nonstick skillet over medium-high heat until crisp, stirring frequently, about 5 minutes. Remove bacon from skillet, drain on paper towels and set aside.

- Sauté onion in bacon drippings until softened, stirring frequently, about 5 minutes. Add garlic and sauté about 1 minute more, stirring constantly.

- Place avocados, lime juice, tomato and sour cream in a medium serving bowl. Add onions with bacon fat to avocado mixture, season to taste with salt, black pepper and cayenne pepper and stir gently to coat.

- Sprinkle bacon and lime zest over avocado salad. Cut tortillas into wedges and serve with the salad. Enjoy!

PER SERVING: Calories: 429; Fat: 34g; Protein: 17g; Carbs: 18g; Fiber: 15g Net Carbs: 3g; Fat 71% / Protein 16% / Carbs 13%

Day 26 Dinner: Butter-Roasted Turkey Breasts

Serves: 4 (plus 2 leftover portions) / Preparation time: 30 minutes / Cooking time: 2 hours

Brushing the turkey breasts underneath the skin allows the flavors to more thoroughly infuse the meat.

2 bone-in turkey breasts (about 6 pounds each)

1/2 cup butter (melted)

4 garlic cloves (minced)

1 tablespoon ground mustard

2 teaspoons dried rosemary (crushed)

2 teaspoons rubbed sage

2 teaspoon dried thyme

2 teaspoons salt

1/2 teaspoon freshly ground black pepper, to taste

2 celery ribs (quartered)

- Preheat oven to 325°F.

- Mix butter, garlic, mustard, rosemary, sage, thyme, salt and pepper. Loosen skin from turkey breasts. Brush turkey breasts with butter mixture and set skin back in place. If any butter mixture remains, brush over turkey skin.

- Arrange celery in the bottom of a large roasting pan and set turkey breasts skin-sides up in pan. Roast turkey, uncovered, until internal temperature reaches 165°F, about 2 hours. If skin is browning too quickly, cover turkey breasts loosely with foil

- When roasting time ends, remove pan from oven, cover loosely with foil and let turkey breasts rest for about 15 minutes. Slice turkey breasts, divide into 3 portions and brush with pan juices. Serve 1 portion of sliced turkey immediately. Let remaining 2 portions cool, cover and refrigerate for later use. Enjoy!

PER SERVING: Calories: 275; Fat: 17g; Protein: 28g; Carbs: 2g; Fiber: 1g Net Carbs: 1g; Fat 56% / Protein 41% / Carbs 3%

Day 27 Breakfast: Smoked Chicken Pockets

Serves: 4 / Preparation time: 10 minutes / Cooking time: 25 minutes

Which came first, the chicken or the egg? It won't matter when you put them together in this savory breakfast treat!

8 eggs (divided)

2 tablespoons butter (divided)

1/4 cup (1 ounce) shredded colby jack cheese

Leftover shredded smoked chicken from Day 22 Dinner

2 tablespoons sour cream

- Crack 2 eggs into a small bowl and beat until thoroughly combined. Melt 1/2 tablespoon butter in a medium nonstick skillet over medium-high heat, add beaten eggs and swirl skillet to coat. Cook eggs until lightly browned on the bottom and nearly cooked through, about 4 minutes. Carefully flip eggs over.

- Sprinkle about 1 tablespoon cheese and about 1/4 of the shredded chicken over half of the cooked eggs and cook until cheese is melted and chicken is heated through. Fold eggs over filling, remove from skillet and keep warm. Repeat with remaining eggs, butter, cheese and chicken.

- Dollop about 1/4 of the sour cream onto each pocket and serve immediately. Enjoy!

PER SERVING: Calories: 353; Fat: 26g; Protein: 27g; Carbs: 2g; Fiber: 0g Net Carbs: 2g; Fat 66% / Protein 31% / Carbs 3%

Day 27 Lunch: Zoodles with Thai Peanut Sauce

Serves: 4 / Preparation time: 15 minutes / Cooking time: 2 minutes

For extra crunch, chop up some roasted peanuts and use as a garnish.

1 leftover portion zoodles from Day 23 Lunch

1/4 cup natural creamy peanut butter

2 tablespoons water

1 tablespoon soy sauce

1 tablespoon coconut oil (melted)

1 garlic clove (minced)

1 tablespoon rice vinegar

1 teaspoon sriracha sauce

1/2 teaspoon ground ginger

1/4 teaspoon sesame oil

- Place zoodles in a colander and let drain while preparing the rest of the recipe.
- Purée peanut butter, water, soy sauce, coconut oil, garlic, rice vinegar, sriracha sauce, ginger and sesame oil in a food processor until smooth
- Transfer zoodles to a large bowl, toss with peanut sauce and heat in the microwave. Serve immediately and enjoy!

PER SERVING: Calories: 202; Fat: 19g; Protein: 6g; Carbs: 6g; Fiber: 2g Net Carbs: 4g; Fat 85% / Protein 12% / Carbs 3%

Day 27 Dinner: Taco Bar

Serves: 4 (plus 2 leftover portions) / Preparation time: 10 minutes / Cooking time: 25 minutes

Cocoa powder and cinnamon lend this ground beef taco filling a deep, dark color and a rich, hearty flavor.

3 pounds ground beef

1 tablespoon garlic powder

1 tablespoon onion powder

1 tablespoon chili powder

1 tablespoon ground cumin

1 tablespoon cocoa powder

1 teaspoon salt, plus more to taste

1 teaspoon freshly ground black pepper, plus more to taste

1/2 teaspoon cayenne pepper, plus more to taste

1/4 teaspoon cinnamon

2 teaspoons dried oregano

4 leftover tortillas from Day 24 Lunch

Taco toppings, such as shredded lettuce, chopped tomatoes, shredded cheese, sour cream, guacamole and sliced olives

- Crumble ground beef in a large nonstick skillet over medium-high heat and cook until browned, stirring frequently, 8 to 10 minutes.

- Add garlic powder, onion powder, chili powder, cumin, cocoa powder, salt, pepper, cayenne pepper and cinnamon and stir until thoroughly combined. Simmer taco filling uncovered until reduced to desired consistency, 5 to 15 minutes, stirring occasionally.

- Add oregano to taco filling and stir until thoroughly combined. Divide taco filling into 3 portions. Assemble a build-your-own-taco bar with one portion filling, the leftover tortillas, and the taco toppings. Let remaining 2 portions of taco filling cool, cover and refrigerate for later use. Enjoy!

PER SERVING (calculated without toppings): Calories: 404; Fat: 32g; Protein: 26g; Carbs: 6g; Fiber: 6g Net Carbs: 0g; Fat 74% / Protein 26% / Carbs 0%

Day 28 Breakfast: Cheesy Bacon Egg Cups

Serves: 4 / Preparation time: 10 minutes / Cooking time: 10 minutes

You can substitute any cheese that melts well for the colby in this recipe. Try Gouda, Swiss, Muenster or Gruyere.

- 2 tablespoons butter
- 1/4 cup heavy cream
- 1/4 cup cream cheese (softened)
- 1/2 cup (2 ounces) grated colby cheese
- 1/4 teaspoon garlic powder
- 1/4 teaspoon onion powder
- Freshly ground black pepper, to taste
- 4 leftover bacon and egg cups from Day 24 Breakfast

- For the sauce, melt butter in a small saucepan over medium heat. Add heavy cream and stir until heated through.

- Add cream cheese to saucepan and stir until melted. Heat mixture to a simmer, stirring frequently. Remove saucepan from heat.

- Add colby cheese, garlic powder, onion powder and pepper and stir until cheese is melted and sauce is creamy.

- Reheat bacon and egg cups in the microwave, drizzle with cheese sauce and serve immediately. Enjoy!

PER SERVING: Calories: 350; Fat: 32g; Protein: 14g; Carbs: 2g; Fiber: 0g Net Carbs: 2g; Fat 82% / Protein 16% / Carbs 2%

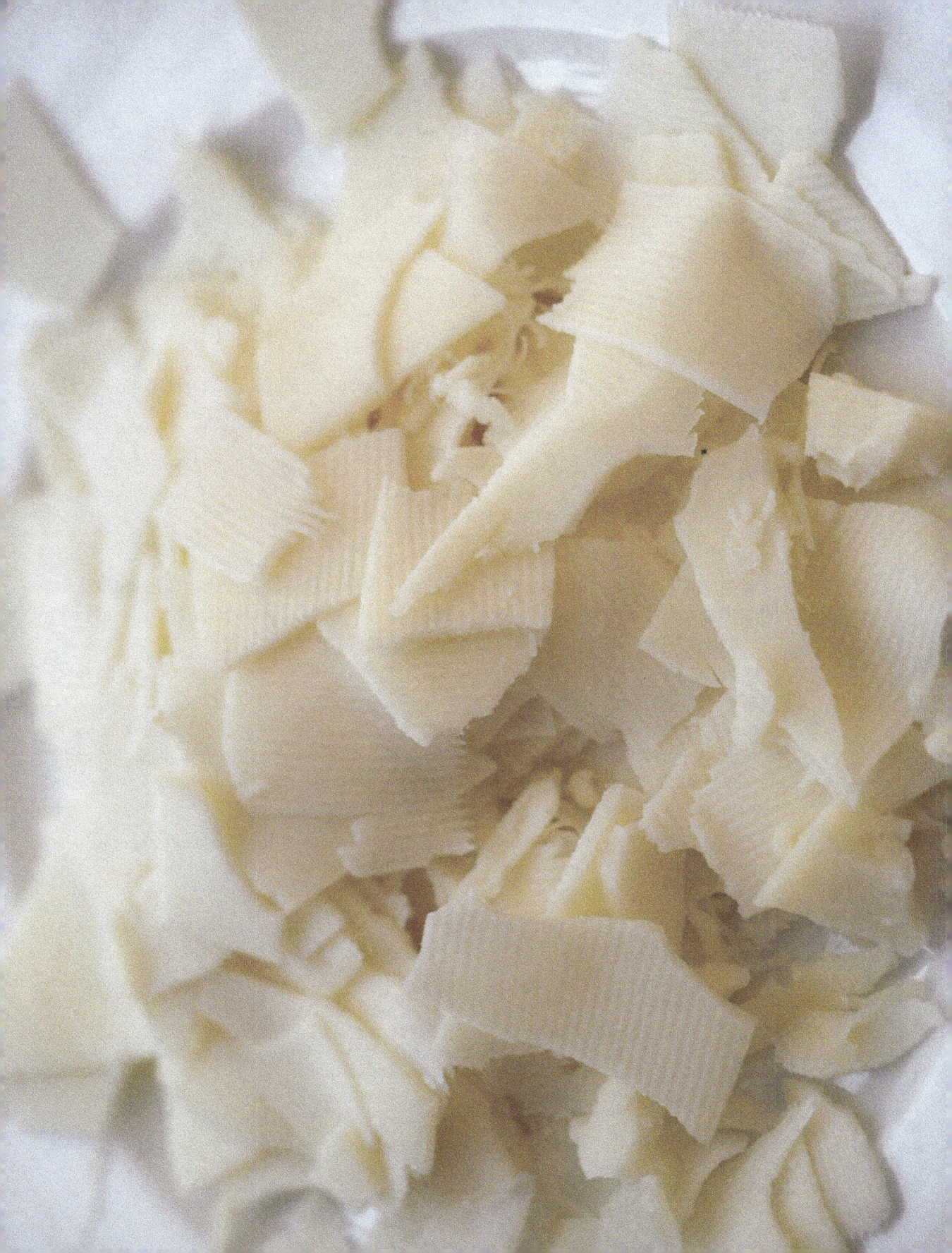

Day 28 Lunch: Eggplant Turkey Lasagna

Serves: 8 / Preparation time: 45 minutes / Cooking time: 45 minutes

This lasagna gives you all the flavors of traditional lasagna, but without the noodles.

1 medium eggplant

2 tablespoons olive oil (divided)

1/2 teaspoon garlic salt

1 small onion (diced)

8 ounces baby bella mushrooms (sliced)

2 garlic cloves (minced)

1 leftover portion turkey breast from Day 26 Dinner (diced)

1 can (8 ounces) tomato sauce

1/2 cup (2 ounces) grated Parmesan cheese

2 teaspoons Italian herb blend

1/4 teaspoon freshly ground black pepper

2 cups (8 ounces) shredded mozzarella cheese

- Preheat oven broiler. Peel eggplant and cut lengthwise into slices about 1/8" thick. Brush slices with 1 tablespoon olive oil and sprinkle with garlic salt. Arrange slices on a baking sheet and broil until tender and lightly browned, 4 to 5 minutes.
- Reduce oven temperature to 350°F. Spray a 13" x 9" casserole dish with nonstick cooking spray and set aside.
- For the sauce, heat remaining 1 tablespoon oil in a large nonstick skillet and sauté onion and mushrooms until softened and lightly browned, 5 to 6 minutes, stirring occasionally. Add garlic and sauté about 1 minute more, stirring constantly. Add turkey, tomato sauce, Parmesan cheese, Italian herb blend and pepper to skillet and stir until combined.
- Layer about 1/3 of the eggplant slices, 1/3 of the sauce and 1/3 of the mozzarella cheese in the prepared casserole dish. Repeat layers with remaining eggplant, sauce and cheese, finishing with cheese on top.
- Bake lasagna until heated through and cheese is melted and golden brown, about 30 minutes. Serve immediately and enjoy!

PER SERVING: Calories: 376; Fat: 23g; Protein: 33g; Carbs: 10g; Fiber: 3g Net Carbs: 7g; Fat 55% / Protein 35% / Carbs 10%

Day 28 Dinner: Grilled Cod Fillets

Serves: 4 (plus 1 leftover portion) / Preparation time: 20 minutes / Cooking time: 10 minutes

These grilled cod fillets would pair nicely with a simple chopped Caprese salad made with fresh sun-ripened tomatoes.

6 cod fillets (8 ounces each)

1/2 teaspoon salt, plus more to taste

1/4 teaspoon freshly ground black pepper, plus more to taste

2 tablespoons butter (melted)

1 lemon (zested, juiced)

3 garlic cloves (minced)

1 teaspoon dried thyme leaves

- Brush grill grate with oil and preheat grill.

- Season cod fillets all over with salt and pepper and set aside.

- For basting, mix butter, lemon juice, garlic and thyme leaves in a small bowl.

- Place cod fillets on grill grates and cook until fillets are flaky and golden brown, about 6 minutes total, basting frequently with butter mixture.

- Remove cod fillets from grill and let stand rest for about 5 minutes. Season fillets to taste with salt and pepper. Sprinkle 4 fillets with lemon zest and serve. Let remaining 2 fillets cool, cover and refrigerate for later use. Enjoy!

PER SERVING: Calories: 304; Fat: 13g; Protein: 41g; Carbs: 4g; Fiber: 0g Net Carbs: 4g; Fat 38% / Protein 54% / Carbs 8%

Day 29 Breakfast: Coconut Almond Bread

Serves: 4 (plus 1 leftover portion) / Preparation time: 40 minutes / Cooking time: 50 to 60 minutes

This dense, nutty-flavored bread is both filling and tasty. It's surprisingly low in carbs, so it's keto-friendly.

1 1/2 cups almond flour

1/3 cup coconut flour

2 tablespoons ground flaxseed

1 1/2 tablespoons psyllium husk powder

Powdered sweetener of choice equal to 1 tablespoon sugar

1 teaspoon baking soda

1/2 teaspoon salt

6 eggs

1 tablespoon butter (melted)

1 tablespoon coconut oil (melted)

1 teaspoon apple cider vinegar

Butter and sugar-free jam, as desired

- Preheat oven to 300°F. Spray an 8" x 4" loaf pan with nonstick cooking spray and set aside.

- In a medium bowl, whisk almond flour, coconut flour, flaxseed, psyllium husk powder, sweetener, baking soda and salt until thoroughly combined. Set dry ingredients aside.

- In a separate bowl, beat eggs with an electric hand mixer until light and frothy, about 3 minutes. Add butter and coconut and beat 1 minute more. Add dry ingredients to egg mixture and beat just until combined. Cover bowl and let batter stand for about 15 minutes.

- Spread batter in prepared pan and bake until bread is golden and tests done with a toothpick, 50 to 60 minutes.

- Remove bread from pan and let cool on a wire rack for 10 minutes. Cut loaf in half and cut one half into slices. Serve sliced bread immediately with butter and sugar-free jam as desired. Let remaining bread cool, place in a paper bag and refrigerate for later use. Enjoy!

PER SERVING: Calories: 243; Fat: 19g; Protein: 10g; Carbs: 8g; Fiber: 5g Net Carbs: 3g; Fat 70% / Protein 16% / Carbs 14%

Day 29 Lunch: Zucchini Enchilada Bake

Serves: 6 / Preparation time: 30 minutes / Cooking time: 30 minutes

If you like cilantro, you can stir some chopped fresh leaves into the dip for this casserole, or sprinkle some over the top before serving.

- 3 medium zucchini (thinly sliced)
- 1 teaspoon salt
- 1 leftover portion taco filling from Day 27 Dinner
- 1 can (14.5 ounces) enchilada sauce
- 2 cups (8 ounces) shredded cheddar cheese
- 1 can (14 ounces) black olives (drained, sliced)
- 1 avocado (pitted, peeled, mashed)
- 1/2 cup sour cream
- 1 Roma tomato (diced)

- Place zucchini slices in a colander, sprinkle with salt and toss to combine. Let zucchini stand for at least 30 minutes.

- Preheat oven to 350°F. Spray a 9" x 13" casserole dish with nonstick cooking spray and set aside.

- Blot zucchini slices dry with paper towels. Layer about 1/3 of the zucchini slices, 1/3 of the taco filling, 1/3 of the sauce, 1/3 of the cheese and 1/3 of the olives. Repeat layers with remaining slices, filling, sauce, cheese and olives, finishing with cheese and olives on the top.

- Bake casserole until cheese is melted and lightly browned, about 30 minutes. Meanwhile, for the dip, mix avocado, sour cream and tomato until thoroughly combined. Serve casserole immediately with the dip and enjoy!

PER SERVING: Calories: 432; Fat: 35g; Protein: 22g; Carbs: 10g; Fiber: 4g Net Carbs: 6g; Fat 73% / Protein 20% / Carbs 7%

Day 29 Dinner: Cucumber Salad with Cod and Basil

Serves: 4 / Preparation time: 20 minutes

For a decorative touch to this salad, peel thin strips from the cucumbers before quartering and cutting. Each piece will then be striped!

4 small fresh cucumbers

2 leftover grilled cod fillets from Day 28 Dinner

1/2 cup fresh basil leaves

3 tablespoons mayonnaise

3 tablespoons low-sugar vinaigrette salad dressing

Salt and freshly ground black pepper, to taste

- Quarter cucumbers lengthwise and remove seeds if desired. Cut cucumbers into bite-size pieces and place in a large serving bowl.
- Flake cod fillets with a fork and add to cucumbers.
- Set aside several basil leaves for garnish. Cut remaining basil leaves into strips, add to cucumbers and cod and toss gently to combine.
- Whisk mayonnaise and vinaigrette, season to taste with salt and pepper and pour over salad. Toss salad gently to coat with dressing. Garnish salad with reserved basil leaves and serve immediately. Enjoy!

PER SERVING: Calories: 285; Fat: 17g; Protein: 22g; Carbs: 10g; Fiber: 3g Net Carbs: 7g; Fat 54% / Protein 31% / Carbs 15%

Day 30 Breakfast: Toast with Almond Butter

Serves: 4 / Preparation time: 10 minutes

The satisfying crunch of toasted bread and nuts pairs perfectly with the creamy nut butter in this hearty and delicious keto-friendly breakfast.

Leftover half loaf of bread from Day 29 Breakfast

2 teaspoons butter

2 tablespoons almond butter

1/4 cup sliced almonds (toasted)

- Cut bread into 8 slices and toast to desired doneness.
- Spread butter and almond butter on toast, sprinkle with almonds and serve immediately. Enjoy!

PER SERVING: Calories: 344; Fat: 28g; Protein: 13g; Carbs: 13g; Fiber: 8g Net Carbs: 5g; Fat 73% / Protein 15% / Carbs 12%

Day 30 Lunch: Turkey Parmesan

Serves: 6 / Preparation time: 30 minutes / Cooking time: 3 to 5 minutes

When preparing the coating, be careful that you don't pulse the mixture for too long. You're aiming for a dry, crumbly mixture.

2 ounces pork rinds

1/4 cup (1 ounce) grated Parmesan cheese

1 teaspoon Italian herb blend

1/4 teaspoon freshly ground black pepper

1/4 cup heavy cream

1 leftover portion turkey breast from Day 26 Dinner

1/2 cup low-sugar marinara sauce

1/2 cup (2 ounces) mozzarella cheese

- Preheat oven broiler. Spray a rimmed baking sheet with nonstick cooking spray.

- For the coating, pulse pork rinds into crumbs in a food processor. Add Parmesan cheese, herb blend and pepper and pulse just until combined. Spread coating in a shallow dish. Pour cream into another shallow dish.

- Dip turkey slices in cream and roll in coating, pressing firmly so coating sticks to slices.

- Arrange coated slices on prepared baking sheet and broil until golden brown, watching closely, 2 to 3 minutes. Flip slices over, top with marinara sauce and cheese and broil until cheese is melted and golden brown, watching closely, 1 to 2 minutes more. Serve immediately and enjoy!

PER SERVING: Calories: 339; Fat: 23g; Protein: 31g; Carbs: 5g; Fiber: 1g Net Carbs: 4g; Fat 61% / Protein 37% / Carbs 2%

Day 30 Dinner: Sloppy José Casserole

Serves: 6 / Preparation time: 15 minutes / Cooking time: 30 minutes

This saucy casserole is reminiscent of sloppy joe filling, but with a decidedly Mexican accent. If you can't find the Mexican cheeses, you can substitute Monterey jack for the queso quesadilla and Parmesan for the Cotija. The casserole will still taste muy bueno.

1 leftover portion taco filling from Day 27 Dinner

1 cup sour cream

1/4 cup heavy cream

1 1/2 cups shredded queso quesadilla (divided)

Canned jalapeño peppers, to taste

2 ounces pork rinds (coarsely crushed)

1/2 cup crumbled Cotija cheese

- Preheat oven to 350°F. Spray a 9" x 13" casserole dish with nonstick cooking spray and set aside.

- In a large bowl, mix taco filling, sour cream, heavy cream, jalapeño peppers and about 1 cup of the queso quesadilla until thoroughly combined. Evenly spread taco filling mixture in prepared casserole dish.

- Sprinkle pork rinds, Cotija cheese and remaining 1/2 cup queso quesadilla over the casserole. Bake casserole until cheeses are melted and casserole is heated through, about 30 minutes. Serve immediately and enjoy!

PER SERVING: Calories: 411; Fat: 32g; Protein: 27g; Carbs: 2g; Fiber: 0g Net Carbs: 2g; Fat 70% / Protein 26% / Carbs 4%

References and Resources

Calton, J. (2010). Prevalence of micronutrient deficiency in popular diet plans. *Journal Of The International Society Of Sports Nutrition*, *7*(1), 24. doi: 10.1186/1550-2783-7-24

Clarke, C. What is the Ketogenic Diet? A Comprehensive Beginner's Guide. Retrieved from https://www.ruled.me/guide-keto-diet/

Dastidar, S. (2017). Sugar, Not Fat, Causes Weight Gain: Professor Of Medicine. Retrieved from https://www.techtimes.com/articles/215934/20171120/sugar-fat-causes-weight-gain-professor-medicine.htm

Fogelholm, M., Anderssen, S., Gunnarsdottir, I., & Lahti-Koski, M. (2012). Dietary macronutrients and food consumption as determinants of long-term weight change in adult populations: a systematic literature review. *Food & Nutrition Research*, *56*(1), 19103. doi: 10.3402/fnr.v56i0.19103

Hallböök, T., Lundgren, J., & Rosén, I. (2007). Ketogenic Diet Improves Sleep Quality in Children with Therapy-resistant Epilepsy. *Epilepsia*, *48*(1). doi: 10.1111/j.1528-1167.2006.00834.x

Kamb, S. The Beginner's Guide to the Keto Diet: Literally Everything You Need to Know. Retrieved from https://www.nerdfitness.com/blog/the-beginners-guide-to-the-keto-diet-or-ketogenic-diet/

Krikorian, R., Shidler, M., Dangelo, K., Couch, S., Benoit, S., & Clegg, D. (2012). Dietary ketosis enhances memory in mild cognitive impairment. *Neurobiology Of Aging*, *33*(2), 425.e19-425.e27. doi: 10.1016/j.neurobiolaging.2010.10.006

Lowery, R., & Wilson, J. (2017). *The Ketogenic Diet: An Authoritative Guide to Ketosis*(1st ed.). Nevada: Victory Belt Publishing.

Moore, J., & Westman, E. (2014). *Keto Clarity: Your Definitive Guide to the Benefits of a Low-Carb, High-Fat Diet* (1st ed.). Nevada: Victory Belt Publishing.

Page, K., Williamson, A., Yu, N., McNay, E., Dzuira, J., McCrimmon, R., & Sherwin, R. (2009). Medium-Chain Fatty Acids Improve Cognitive Function in Intensively Treated Type 1 Diabetic Patients and Support In Vitro Synaptic Transmission During Acute Hypoglycemia. *Diabetes*, *58*(5), 1237-1244. doi: 10.2337/db08-1557

Paoli, A. (2014). Ketogenic Diet for Obesity: Friend or Foe?. *International Journal Of*

Environmental Research And Public Health, *11*(2), 2092-2107. Doi: 10.3390/ijerph110202092

Paoli, A., Rubini, A., Volek, J., & Grimaldi, K. (2013). Beyond weight loss: a review of the therapeutic uses of very-low-carbohydrate (ketogenic) diets. *European Journal Of Clinical Nutrition*, *67*(8), 789-796. doi: 10.1038/ejcn.2013.116

Phinney, S., Bistrian, B., Evans, W., Gervino, E., & Blackburn, G. (1983). The human metabolic response to chronic ketosis without caloric restriction: Preservation of submaximal exercise capability with reduced carbohydrate oxidation. *Metabolism*, *32*(8), 769-776. doi: 10.1016/0026-0495(83)90106-3

Rogawski, M., Löscher, W., & Rho, J. (2016). Mechanisms of Action of Antiseizure Drugs and the Ketogenic Diet. *Cold Spring Harbor Perspectives In Medicine*, *6*(5), a022780. doi: 10.1101/cshperspect.a022780

Titlow, M. (2017). The Definitive Guide to Micronutrients in the Keto Diet. Retrieved from https://www.compoundsolutions.com/news/micronutrients-in-the-ketogenic-diet

Volek, J., Phinney, S., Kossoff, E., Eberstein, J., & Moore, J. (2011). *The art and science of low carbohydrate living*. Lexington, Ky.: Beyond Obesity.

Zajac, A., Poprzecki, S., Maszczyk, A., Czuba, M., Michalczyk, M., & Zydek, G. (2014). The Effects of a Ketogenic Diet on Exercise Metabolism and Physical Performance in Off-Road Cyclists. *Nutrients*, *6*(7), 2493-2508. doi: 10.3390/nu6072493

INDEX

A

Asparagus Mimosa, 93
Avocado Egg Salad Wraps, 88
Avocado Salad, 125

B

Bacon and Egg Cups, 118
Bacon Cheddar Sandwiches, 103
Bacon Cheddar Scramble, 73
Bacon Mushroom Crepes, 56
Bacon-Wrapped Sausage, 96
BBQ Meatballs, 117
Beef with Zoodles, 64
Berries and Cream Pancakes, 111
Broccoli Beef Alfredo, 71
Brunch Meat Loaf, 83
Butter Roasted Turkey Breasts, 126
Buttered Zoodles, 116

C

Cashew Pork Stir Fry, 65
Cheeseburger Salad, 51
Cheesy Bacon Egg Cups, 130
Chicken Breasts with Lemon Dill Butter, 69
Chicken Cordon Bleu Casserole, 72
Chicken Taco Bowls, 52
Chicken Tikka Masala, 59
Chocolate Almond Smoothies, 108
Chorizo Crepes, 44
Cinnamon Roll Pancakes, 53
Coconut Almond Bread, 134
Country-Style Ribs, 94
Creamy White Chili, 98
Cucumber Salad with Cod and Basil, 136
Curry Deviled Eggs, 90

E

Egg and Sausage Bake, 63
Egg Bites with Bacon, 77
Egg Yolk Frittata, 123
Eggplant Turkey Lasagna, 132

G

Garlic Shrimp Zoodles Alfredo, 122
Green Smoothies, 114
Grilled Burgers, 75
Grilled Cheese Sandwiches, 97
Grilled Cod Fillets, 133
Grilled Salmon, 45

H

Ham & Swiss Frittata, 80
Ham and Cheddar Crepes, 74
Ham and Swiss Panini, 109
Ham Roll-Ups, 68
Hoisin Burgers, 91

K

Kale Pesto Tilapia, 112
Keto Almond Pancakes, 47
Keto Coconut Pancakes, 99
Keto Quesadilla, 119
Keto Vanilla Yogurt, 102

L

Lemon Butter Tilapia, 100

M

Meatball Parmigiana, 104
Meatball Stroganoff, 110
Mediterranean-Style Salmon, 49

N

Nutty Swiss Bites, 87

P

Pancakes with Peanut Butter Fluff, 105
Pesto Chicken, 78
Pizza Burgers, 82
Pork "Egg Roll" Bowls, 54
Pork Medallions, 48
Pulled Pork, 101

R

Raspberry Cheesecake Smoothies, 66
Raspberry Pancakes, 60
Roasted Chicken, 46

S

Salmon Patties, 55
Sausage, Egg & Cheese Slices, 86
Savory Spinach Crepes, 50
Shredded Pork Taco Salads, 107
Sloppy José Casserole, 139

Slow Cooker Pulled Ham, 62
Smoked Chicken Pockets, 127
Smoky Chicken Soup, 120
Smoky Slow Cooker Chicken, 113
Spinach and Salmon Salad with Strawberry Vinaigrette, 61
Spinach Frittata with Bacon, 92
Strawberry Cheesecake Smoothies, 121
Stuffed Green Peppers, 58

T

Taco Bar, 129
Tilapia Cakes, 106
Toast with Almond Butter, 137
Tuna Salad, 84
Turkey Parmesan, 138
Turkey Skillet, 89
Turkey Zucchini Boats, 85
Tzatziki Eggs, 76

V

Veggie Bacon Egg Cups, 124

W

Wilted Spinach Salad, 81

Z

Zoodles with Thai Peanut Sauce, 128
Zucchini and Onion Eggs, 70
Zucchini Enchilada Bake, 135

www.ingramcontent.com/pod-product-compliance
Lightning Source LLC
Chambersburg PA
CBHW081507080526
44589CB00017B/2682